The *Bad*Kitty

Handbook

A Journey Toward *Authentic*

Female Sensuality

Lisa
Enjoy Your Journey !
♡ Christie ☺
Meow !

by Christie Mawer

The Bad Kitty Handbook
Journey Towards Authentic Female Sensuality

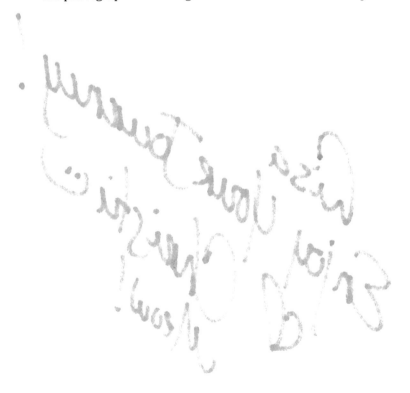

ISBN: 978-0-9825755-7-4
Published and printed by Motivational Press

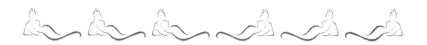

MORE PRAISE FOR THE BAD KITTY HANDBOOK

"I felt connected with Christie and her experiences in this book. She made me realize that there are things I can do to make my life more expressive and sensual. I look forward to taking the gifts Christie has given me in her book and pass them onto my two beautiful daughters so they can have more vibrant and fulfilling lives. Christie and her message is inspiring and her work is transformational for women of all ages."
—*Kim Deep, Edmonton*

"In The Bad Kitty Handbook, Christie shows, through her own story, how much vision and courage it takes to pursue your dreams and to follow your heart. Her journey to find her true calling was not so different from my own. My experiences have shown me that the struggle to validate my choice to be a professional artist is far outweighed by the absolute joy that comes from making a living doing what I love. Christie reminds me that one of the greatest joys in life comes from simply being myself."
—*Janice Blaine, Calgary*

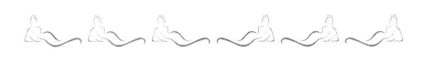

THE BAD KITTY EXPRESSES

HER GRATITUDE:

To all my fabulous and encouraging friends who helped me get to this point, especially the gorgeous members of my Mastermind Group who have kept me accountable and my wonderful and patient designer. To all the wonderful women I have worked with ove the years that have taught me so much and allowed me to pass what I've learned onto them so openly.

To every woman who wants to learn, grow and play! To the universe for teaching me the lessons I needed to get to this place.

CONTENTS:

HOW TO USE THIS BOOK

INTRODUCTION

HOW TO USE THIS BOOK:

This book is a journey and every journey requires a road map. Even with a map, you can go along blindly barely remembering the journey once you arrive at your destination. Or you can enjoy every little moment along the way, arriving enlightened and changed by the experience.

In order to complete the journey of THE BAD KITTY HANDBOOK enlightened, here are a few tips.

There are a few sections in every chapter called BAD KITTY SCRATCHING POST. These are activities for you to do to sharpen your claws and make discoveries on your journey. DO THESE! Do them when they come up. It's important to experience things in the moment rather than putting them off.

The following trip tips will help you to complete your journey without getting lost.
- Each chapter is followed by several blank pages. Use these for your notes and written exercises.
- Go through the book with a friend. Keep each other accountable and share your insights with each other.
- Hire Christie as your coach as you go through the book. She will keep you accountable, be able to answer any of your questions and give you deeper insights into your personal discoveries.

And most of all have fun! Enjoy the journey. The destination will come; the journey is not to be missed.

INTRODUCTION:

Welcome ladies and curious gentlemen. Thank you so much for stopping by and picking up the BAD KITTY HANDBOOK. I'm sure many of you already have some ideas on what the title means. I'm sure some of you were titillated and that's why you picked it up – especially you naughty boys – love you all!

Let me fill you in as to what you can expect from THE BAD KITTY HANDBOOK.

Have you ever looked at someone else and thought – wow, she sure has it all together, how does she do that? Or – wow, everyone seems to really like her, why? Or – wow, I wish I could be like that, what does she have that I don't?

Have you ever met someone who had the qualities just mentioned, but when you got to know them you found many chinks in their armour? They are the actors among us; the over-compensators. The ones who have low confidence so they cover it over with a big act. They are always flushed out eventually. There is that nagging feeling you get when you talk to them that something isn't quite right. They know you will find out the truth at some point, and they are fearful and you can feel that fear.

You may have even been one of the actors at one time – or still are. You have felt that fear of discovery. You have wished that you could be truly confident and have it all together but you just don't know how.

There are many others out there who I call BAD KITTIES who are truly confident, sure of themselves and comfortable in their own skin. They are open, loving, caring people who are unafraid to express their true selves. They stand out in a crowd whether they are extroverts or wall flowers. There is an essence that makes them visible and attractive no matter what their outward appearance.

What separates the poser, the wisher and the true BAD KITTY is AUTHENTIC SENSUALITY. Wait, wait, wait! Did she just say SEXuality? No, read it again – SENSuality. Yes, there is a difference. They are connected in some ways, but in the larger sense, they are not the same.

In this book we will discover the true meaning of Authentic Sensuality which will help you be a BAD KITTY. We will discuss the difference between Sensuality and Sexuality. We will uncover the secrets of how to fully express your personal Sensuality. I will give you tips on how to be truly in touch with your environment, inside and out, fully engaged with your senses, inside and out, and therefore, be fully Sensual. We will talk about what it really means to be a BAD KITTY.

- Have you wanted to stand out in a crowd but thought you were too insignificant or not interesting or unique enough to do so? Being a BAD KITTY will give you that.

- Have you lost touch with who you are? Being a BAD KITTY will give you yourself.

- Have you forgotten your dreams and ambitions? Being a BAD KITTY will reignite them.

- Do you want more confidence? Being a BAD KITTY is confidence.

- Are you completely burned out? Being a BAD KITTY will stoke the fire.

- Do you think you are undesirable or unloved? Being a BAD KITTY will open your heart to a myriad of possibilities.

- Are you doing things that don't work for you simply because you can't say no? Being a BAD KITTY will give you strength of will.

Big claims? Yes. Possible? Absolutely!

Through personal experience and the experience of people I have worked with, I can assure you that true and full expression of your Authentic Sensuality and owning your BAD KITTY will give you these goodies and so many more!

BAD KITTIES truly love themselves. Authentic Sensuality is seeing what you may have considered flaws in the past and loving them because they are part of what makes you so incredible. Authentic Sensuality is seeing that you ARE incredible! We are all amazing, fabulous creatures. Many of us have decided to take on what others have said about us in the past, usually due to their own insecurities, and make them our truth. This has squashed your BAD KITTY.

I'm here to tell you that the truth is: YOU'RE BEAUTIFUL! Every inch of you inside and out - no matter your size, shape or personality - is Beautiful.

- Did someone tell you that you had a big butt? What if you own that big beautiful bootie?

- Did someone tell you that you were too loud?

What if you spoke up anyway?

- Did someone tell you that you were too fat? What if you love those curves?

- Did someone tell you that you weren't smart? What if the truth was that you made them feel stupid?

- Did someone tell you that you couldn't dance? What if you dance with abandon anyway?

- Did someone tell you that you would never succeed? What if your definition of success is different from theirs?

- Did someone tell you that you had a big nose? What if they had a small face?

- Did someone tell you that your dream was impossible? What if Edison, Franklin, Columbus and a myriad of others had listened to the nay-sayers?

The ultimate purpose of this book is for you to see things differently. It is for you to see yourself and your surroundings in a new light. You will use your Authentic Sensuality to feel new sensations in old situations. You will look in the mirror and see a new face. Your perception of everything around you will be altered. You will proudly own and express your BAD KITTY.

The one thing I wish for you all, dear readers, is that you BE BEAUTIFUL, BE YOU. Be your true Authentically Sensual selves and show your BAD

KITTY off to the world. We've been waiting long enough to see it. Quit hiding and get out there, you gorgeous thing you!

Now turn the page and get started!

CHAPTER ONE: THE BAD KITTY REVEALED

THE BAD KITTY'S TAIL:

Once upon a time I was a little girl. Actually, I was never very little. I've always been tall. I wasn't one of those kids who were small or even average and then one day had a growth spurt. All through school I was the kid in the middle of the back row of the school pictures and at the back of the room so that I wouldn't block anyone's view.

I was never small and I never wanted to be a girl. I wished and wished I was a boy. It appeared to me that boys were stronger; more respected and had better lives overall than we put-upon girls. It wasn't fair, so rather than being a weak, insignificant girl, I tried to be more like the boys.

One example of how girls were perceived to be less than boys came in Grade 3. My teacher was Mrs. Horseman, my favourite teacher in the school. I loved her because she was tall, beautiful, nice, and creative and she had the word Horse in her name. We were reading a book about Mr. Mugs, the big shaggy sheepdog, going into space. We built a spaceship as part of the process. When we were done with that section, she asked who would like to take the spaceship home. A boy – who I had a crush on – and I both put up our hands so she asked us to pick a number between 1 and 10. I was closest and was so excited. Then Mrs.Horseman crushed my world and my opinion of her and, I'm sure, many persons of authority to come, by saying, "I'm going to give it to Mark because this is more a boy's toy."

That clinched it. Being a girl sucked!

Right around that time, my parents also divorced. In the early 70's, divorce was much more of a rarity than it is now. My sister and I were the odd kids out and many teachers made a point of taking notice of that. I know they were trying to be helpful, but it really had the opposite effect.

As the oldest child of a broken home who hated being a girl and who was constantly told how strong she was by her mother, I denied my femininity in order to be more like a man. I had to be the strong one. I couldn't show my feelings.

I had to live up to expectations. I apparently did a fabulous job as my sister used to call me Spock.

A number of things also contributed to my learning to be invisible; always being in the back certainly helped. Even though I could see over everyone else, I was the lonely one hiding in behind. We moved a lot, so I got really good at blending into whatever new situation and school we were put into. My sister was the pretty and outgoing one and got all the attention. I usually let her make friends in a new place and I'd be the tag-along. And, yes, you read right earlier, I was the oldest but I was the hanger-on. I am smart but I only did just enough so that I would be high to middle of the road, not the best, so I wouldn't have the pressure.

Oddly, though, I wanted to stand out. There were times when I was chosen out of the crowd and it felt so great, but I couldn't handle it and would do something to sabotage it.

In grade 6 another favourite teacher, Mrs. Noble, saw beyond my shell. She saw the star hiding inside. She chose me to have speaking parts in plays. Up until then no one saw my acting aspirations and there was no way I would ever have said anything to them about it. She gave me an award for a picture I had drawn and then asked me to teach the class how to draw a horse. She was my hero.

Our mom went away for some work training and left a college girl to look after us. One day she skipped school, something I didn't know you could do, and my sister and I got inspired and stayed home for a week. We got caught, of course, and when I saw the disappointment on my favourite teacher's face, it broke my heart. I didn't know until much later that what I had done was a subconscious way of removing expectations so I wouldn't have to live up to them.

For many years I lived in this state of trying to be something I wasn't; trying to be a boy, trying to be invisible. Trying to be what I thought others wanted me to be. And, of course, I was miserable.

In my 30's I started to discover and reinstate my true self. It certainly wasn't an overnight process. It's still happening, actually, but eventually The BAD KITTY, my authentic self, re-emerged.

I have a passion to help people. First I was going to teach Self Esteem to teens. Then the man who was to become my coach, Andrew Barber Starkey, pointed out that what I'm really all about is Self Expression, "look at your hair, the way you dress, everything about you is about expression." And, as he has been many times since, he was totally right.

I still thought I was meant to teach teens. I went on that path for a bit with limited success. I did make an impact on some, but I was having trouble creating the vision I had because I wasn't all that clear on what it was.

WHERE THE BAD KITTY CAME FROM:

Then the relationship I had when this journey began ended, adding more pieces to the growth equation. One big piece was discovering pole dancing parties. That became my business. I loved it; it suited my fun and performance-loving personality, and I saw something very interesting happen. I saw women come alive. They were just dancing with a piece of vertical stainless steel, but it made a huge difference in their self perception in such a short time.

That got me thinking about what it meant and how I could expand on it. The term Sensuality Coach came to me. I used it for over a year. I was teaching women to be more sensual. Slowly, a new business started to form. Bits and pieces came to me over time.

As with anything, it didn't really start to come together until I started to seriously work on it. I created my blog accessible from my main website - www.thebadkitty.com, started work on the website and on this book. As I worked on it, a key was still missing. It was safe and nice and I had to explain a lot to get people to understand. Still, I was left with a lot of, "uh huh, that's nice" kind of reactions.

Then I met Berny Dohrman. I met with him for only a moment and he completely got me, got what I wanted to do and branded me as THE BAD KITTY.

I loved it. It rang with my soul and my personality, but I still resisted – for a moment. I realized that this was the part that was missing on so many levels. THE BAD KITTY has an edge and a hint of sex. I have an edge and more than a hint of sex. It draws people in. When he said it at the meeting, everyone else there lit up. It leaves room for growth into many arenas. It's fun. Cats are extremely sensual creatures. It's perfect! Wouldn't we all love to lounge around all day being stroked? I have three cats of my own and boy they have a good life.

Having THE BAD KITTY brand put a new spin on what I was doing and solidified everything. Granted, I had to get the domain THE BAD KITTY.com as BAD KITTY.com was already taken by a porn site. And, yes, it does bring that image to some minds – you naughty boys, for example, if you're still reading. And I like that aspect of it. A little controversy gets people involved.

THE BAD KITTY REVEALED:

Have you ever had a cat? Known someone who had a cat or been around cats? If you have – and I'm pretty sure that covers everyone – you know that cats have a mind of their own. As humans, we have certain expectations of our cats. We want them to behave in a certain way. When they don't behave according to our expectations; they scratch our favourite chair, eat the plants, take a ride on the curtains – we get upset. We spray them with water and call them "bad cat". In reality, they are just being their natural kitty selves. It's not really good or bad, it simply is the way they are.

So it is with us. We are born perfect. And we live in a society with people that have certain expectations of us. We are told by everyone around us how we "should" be. We get so many messages from so many people that we try to live up to. Being a Bad Kitty is about reclaiming the things that we've set aside about ourselves in order to be more acceptable to those around us. Unfortunately it never really works, there are still those who are disappointed. So why not reclaim your Bad Kitty self. When you do, you will experience a difference in your life in subtle, and not so subtle, ways.

A BAD KITTY is someone who:
- knows who she is
- is in touch with all aspects of herself, including her sexuality (ahem, where's your mind?)
- is unafraid to express herself
- loves being a girl (which has a wide definition, as we will discover)
- knows the power of being a girl
- refuses to be invisible
- creates her dreams
- loves herself (no, not that way – well, not only that way...)
- knows that by being true to herself, she has more to give the others in her life
- is open hearted
- is unstoppable
- lives in the moment
- stands up for herself
- knows what she wants
- has a zest for life
- makes a positive impact

In essence, a BAD KITTY is a true, honest and complete woman. She is expressing herself, which makes her Sensual. She is fully engaged in all aspects of life from sights, sounds and smells to sex. Others are drawn to her. She is open and no one can resist true, open Authentic Sensuality. It is inspiring! Every woman is a BAD KITTY under-neath all the expectations and standards imposed by others. All it takes is the willingness to let go of those expectations and standards so you can BE BEAUTIFUL, BE YOU.

BAD KITTY SCRATCHING POST:

Get a pen and paper and set it near you (or use the empty pages at the end of the chapter). Sit quietly. Breathe deeply. Think back to your youth. Feel the endless possibilities and dreams that you had when you were younger. Nothing was impos-sible. The world was waiting for you to conquer it. There were no obstacles, no responsibilities – only possibilities. Your heart was open. Your emotions flowed freely. You loved with abandon. You cried until all the sadness was gone. You screamed loudly when you were angry so that everyone knew and you could release the energy. You laughed with full and complete joy.

Go back to this place. Let it wash over you. Imagine you can carry those feelings into the here and now. Feel the power that it gives you and the inspiration that washes over you.

Recall your dreams. Some may no longer be valid. Your desires may have changed. Remember the energy the dreams gave you, whether they still speak to you or not. Feel the thrill of discovery and potential. Now take that feeling into now. What are your big dreams? If nothing was holding you back, what would you do? If no one had expectations of you, what would you do? If you were completely free to do what drives you, what would it be?

Let those thoughts come to you uncensored. Put the obstacles aside. There are none in your dream world. The road is clear and all obstacles become stepping stones. What sensations do you feel? Is your energy rising? Is your stomach getting butter-flies? Are you smiling?

Slowly come back to the room you are in. Breathe deeply and hold onto the energy and positive sensations you have just experienced.

Take the pen and paper and write down your thoughts, feelings, sensations and especially the dreams that came to you. Write uncensored. Let it flow.

THE MARTYR COMPLEX:

These feelings and dreams you have just experienced are part of your BAD KITTY self. As women, we tend to be martyrs. There is an expectation in our society that women are to be caregivers. Men do the fighting, we do the healing. Basically, this is true. Women are the "softer" sex and it is in our nature to nurture.

The problem comes when our care-giving nature overtakes everything else. This is when the martyr raises its head. The martyr is the woman who has forgotten that she is important, too. The martyr has forgotten, or doesn't realize, that in order to give to others she has to take care of herself first. The martyr is running on empty in her energy levels and joy levels. The martyr is slowly killing herself – who she is, her BAD KITTY - from the inside.

THE BAD KITTY'S TAIL:

I used to be married. It seems like a million years ago. I was a totally different person then; a person who didn't know herself.

I was a church-going gal back then. Religion, church and all that goes with it is not bad. I have great respect for those who believe and work in integrity in that life. For me, it created a lot of pressure. Part of that pressure was around sex. I take after my mother – I have a much higher sex drive than most women. I felt pressure to find a decent man and get married so that I could have sex without guilt. I didn't succeed in the "no sex before marriage" and had buckets of guilt on my shoulders because of it. Rather than motivating me to purity and self love, it made me despise me and what I perceived at that time to be weakness.

When I met a nice man who loved me – or so we both thought in our naive youth – who wanted to be a youth pastor, I thought I had hit pay dirt. We got married roughly a year after we started dating.

It wasn't long before things started to go wrong. We were too young. We didn't know what we wanted in life. We both tried to push the other to be who we expected them to be rather than supporting each other to be who we were. Eventually things broke down completely and we divorced. He has gone on, from all reports, to be very happy and fulfilled in his chosen life, as have I.

Being a wife was being a martyr for me. He was the "important" one. My job was to support him no matter what. It was killing me. I didn't know it at the time, as I wasn't clear on what I needed in life. Based on the anger that was raging through me nearly every day at the end, it became clear I wasn't where I needed to be.

A friend once said that I was a "good wife". The truth is I was good at *pretending* to be a good wife. I knew what was expected and I did it. After the divorce I realized that that role did not work for me. I'm far too independent. I support my friends and family. I love to do what I can to help out. However, the daily expectation of cooking meals, cleaning up and making my husband feel good was not for me.

The martyr can sneak in so easily. One great check-in to see if you are in martyr mode is to look at your dreams. Do they revolve around others? Is there anything completely selfish in there?

ANOTHER BAD KITTY'S TAIL:

I did a workshop recently where I asked the women to talk about their big dreams. The first woman, Jennifer* (all names have been changed unless express permission has been given), had a hard time coming up with a dream. The women in the workshop knew each other well so they prompted Jennifer with some things they had heard her speak about. Finally she came up with the fact that she wanted to create a CD of her music. That's huge!

Several of the other women in that same work-shop had the dream of "creating a strong family who loves each other". There is nothing inherently wrong with this dream. We all want our families to be loving and strong. The red flag for me is that they couldn't come up with something that had nothing to do with their family. How can you give to your family if you have nothing special for yourself? What kind of example are you setting for your children if you are continually giving and never receiving?

BAD KITTY SCRATCHING POST:

Go back over the dreams you wrote down earlier. Make an itemized list if you did not do so earlier.

Do you have some that revolve around others?

"Buy my mom a nice house". "Make enough money to send my kids to a good university." "Spend more time with my family." "Buy Christmas gifts earlier and with more thought." Mark all of these dreams with an O (as in others).

The remaining dreams should revolve around you. "Go skydiving." "Write a book." "Go for a walk everyday." "Scrapbook." "Have a girl's night."

Cross out all the ones that don't fall into either of these categories, if any.

Count how many O dreams you have. Do they outnumber the unmarked ones? If so, you are running in martyr mode.

Take a few minutes and see how many purely selfish goals you can come up with. If you have trouble thinking of any, you are in deep martyr mode!

BAD KITTIES know how to have a balanced life. They know that in order to make the O dreams come true they have to work on some of the selfish ones as well.

BAD KITTY SCRATCHING POST:

Choose one selfish dream you want to accomplish in the next 6 months. Circle it. Write it on an index card and put it somewhere you will see it every day – in your office, on your bathroom mirror, on the fridge. Create small steps in order to make this dream a reality. As you work towards it, notice how your energy level and attitude change in your life as a whole.

In order to BE BEAUTIFUL, BE YOU, you need to know yourself. You need to know what makes you a BAD KITTY. You need to own your dreams!

We're going to work on it. Let's continue on the journey.

CHAPTER TWO:

I'M NOT SURE I WANT TO BE A BAD KITTY

I've run into objections to this chapter title on a couple of occasions. So let's review the definition of a BAD KITTY from Chapter One.

A BAD KITTY is someone who:
- knows who she is
- is in touch with all aspects of herself, including her sexuality
- is unafraid to express herself
- loves being a girl
- knows the power of being a girl
- refuses to be invisible
- creates her dreams
- loves herself
- knows that by being true to herself, she has more to give the others in her life
- is open hearted
- is unstoppable
- lives in the moment
- stands up for herself
- takes time to smell the roses
- knows what she wants
- has a zest for life
- makes a positive impact

Is there honestly anything in there that you don't want? There may be some of the definitions that give you a bit of a hitch in your stomach. Is that because you don't want it or because you deep down want it so badly and have become so far removed from it that it scares you to go there? Be honest, you want to be more of a BAD KITTY!

COMFORT ZONE:

We all have a Comfort Zone. This is the wall we put around us that says "I can do this, but not that", "I'll go here, but not there", "I enjoy doing this but not that", "I'm good at this, but suck at that", "This is moral, this is wrong." There is nothing inherently

wrong with having a Comfort Zone. Where the problem lies is when it becomes limiting.

If there is something that you really want to have, be or achieve and you feel discomfort around the thought of getting or creating it in your life, you need to break free of that Comfort Zone. It can be difficult. It will be uncomfortable. AT FIRST. Once you do things a few times, it gets more and more comfortable and before you know it, it becomes part of who you are and your Comfort Zone has expanded.

THE BAD KITTY'S TAIL:

All my life I labelled myself as someone who couldn't sell. I would say, "I couldn't sell heaters to Eskimos." I had a belief that sales were beyond me. That there was a type of person that was good at sales – usually pushy and obnoxious – which just wasn't me.

I worked at Sears for a number of years and part of the job was to "sell" the credit card. I was complaining to a friend about having to do this and how much I hated it and she said, "You're an actress, why don't you just pretend you're good at it?"

Sometimes our friends are so smart! I did just that and suddenly I started to get results. Soon I didn't even have to pretend, asking became second nature and no's weren't as likely to deter me from continuing.

A few years later my coach told me that in order to become the person I wanted with a business, I needed to get out there and do sales. All businesses require sales whether you are selling yourself, your idea or a product.

I ended up working for my brother in law. Either he saw something in me or he just didn't want to put an ad in the paper. Whatever the case, I started doing sales for him. In the first year I did all his sales and we sold over $500,000 of Cabinet Refacing. The following year we hired a second sales person and I was doing half as many locations. My sales remained nearly the same as the previous year with half as much territory. The next year I cut back even further and maintained my levels once again. In addition, one of my locations which had been second last in sales in previous years was now number one of 10 in the city and number 7 of 100s in the country!

These experiences gave me the confidence and skills to go forward in creating THE BAD KITTY and to know that if there is something that I haven't done before or am uncomfortable with; I can push myself through that barrier and find a way. I will network, talk about myself, ask for the sale or an action and all with a sense of being grounded and of comfort I wouldn't have had without pushing myself to sell.

And, by the way, I rock now!

BAD KITTY SCRATCHING POST:

Sometime this next week, find something that scares you. Be aware of challenges that come your way. It could be something fairly small, like asking a hard question, or something huge, like changing the direction of your career.

Whatever it is, there should be a feeling of constriction, of "that's not me" or "I can't do it". In addition to that, there will be a feeling of desire and a pull to do it anyway. The voices of "can't" will come from your head. The feeling of can will come from your gut, your heart. There will be a deep knowing despite the voice.

That little voice needs to be acknowledged. Make a decision to follow your heart and gut and say to your little voice, the Saboteur, "Thank you for sharing, I'm up to something else." And keep saying it every timc the constricting thoughts come in.

Then do it! Do the thing that scares you. How did it feel? Notice how much easier it is to do the next time the voice comes up. Keep at it every time there is a conflict between your head and your heart.

STANDARDS:

Part of the difficulty in owning your full self, your Authentic Sensuality, your BAD KITTY-ness, is that we have, over time, forgotten or covered over parts of ourselves. We have been told that something we want is wrong or impossible. We have been directed in a way that someone else thought was right for us and, because we respected them or didn't know any better, we listened.

Most of this comes from adopting the standards of others. Those others are usually people of authority: parents, teachers, religious leaders. Or it could be from peer pressure. Either way, we have looked to others and thought, they must be right and I must be wrong so I'll change.

Everyone is perfect the way they were made. We were all born with dreams and passions and a way of being that was perfect. We all know what is best for ourselves. We all know what makes us happiest. Unfortunately, many of us have forgotten it or buried it so deep we don't know where to find it.

THE BAD KITTY'S TAIL:

When I was a girl, I wanted to be a performer more than anything. I wanted to be famous. I didn't care if it was for acting or singing – or both. I just wanted to be out there: noticed and loved. I was always writing plays for me and my sister to perform. I would lip synch with my mom's Neil Diamond and Pet Clark records. Oh my, am I dating myself. How many of you reading this even know who those people are? Or have used a record player? Deep breath ... O.K....

I would create dance routines. My favourite games involved pretend. One of my favourites was to gallop around the house as a horse. My jeans always had holes in the knees!

I remember a moment when things started to shift. I was in Grade 5. We were living up north in a small city called Grande Prairie. My parents had been divorced for a couple of years and my sister and I had been uprooted from Regina, where we had been all of our short lives.

I rebelled in small ways when we lived in the trailer outside of town. I would refuse to go on car trips. I would have temper tantrums in my room at the slightest provocation. I would refuse to practice the piano or do my homework. In retrospect, I was not happy with the turn my life had taken.

One time, when everyone else had headed off for a drive in the country, I stayed home and danced. I created something to the song *Age of Aquarius* – I'm an Aquarian - that I thought was wonderful. I worked on it over and over and felt fabulous about my creation. When the family came home, I showed it to them.

Rather than applause or even a simple "nice job" I got a patronizing look and "What did you do that for?" That may not be the exact wording of the response, but that was the feeling I got from it. In that moment I shrank. My BAD KITTY lost a lot of steam and began to live in fear of ridicule.

BAD KITTY SCRATCHING POST:

Take a moment to sit quietly. Close your eyes and go back in time. Look for moments where you lost a piece of yourself. Look for times when you felt belittled. Find the times when you felt unheard or unappreciated. I'm sure you can find at least a few.

Go into that moment. Really feel it. Allow your-self to experience it again. See it with your new adult eyes and feel it with your younger, in the moment, self.

Journal your memories and feelings of the

experience.

These events have helped shape who you are now. They have also helped deplete or even eliminate your BAD KITTY. If the description of the BAD KITTY at the top of the chapter gives you feelings of longing or fear, we have some work to do.

- Do you want to do important things in your life?

- Do you want to make an impact in the lives of others?

- Do you want to live a joyful, fulfilled life?

- Do you want to create a legacy?

- Do you want to feel and be present every day?

- Do you want to be confident in your life?

- Do you have dreams that you want to accomplish?

Then you want to regain your AUTHENTIC SENSUALITY and live as a BAD KITTY.

SENSUALITY REVEALED:

It's time to understand what AUTHENTIC SENSUALITY is.

Our society has mixed SENSUALITY and SEXUALITY up. They are often used interchangeably. I can't begin to count how many times I have told someone about what I do and have had them misunderstand. I've had many people in conversation say something along the lines of "when you teach women about their SEXuality..." Or several times at networking events I've had women who help other women with problems with sex or their cycles or other genital related issues come up to discuss doing joint ventures. Not that I'm against that by any stretch; it simply shows how closely interlinked the two words have become in our minds.

The definition of SENSUALITY has changed over the centuries. In the 1300's it was:
"part of man that is concerned with the senses" or the "capacity for sensation" and "endowed with feeling, sensitive". (*Online Etymology Dictionary,* © *2001 Douglas Harper*)

By the 1600's it had changed to:
"animal instincts and appetites", "the lower nature regarded as a source of evil, lusts of the flesh". (*Online Etymology Dictionary,* © *2001 Douglas Harper*)

Many things happened in those 300 years that changed society in general and facilitated this change. The 1300s and 1400s were a time of growth and openness. This was the first instance of the Renaissance. Incredibly creative minds like Michelangelo, Dante and Petrarch abounded. New philosophies such as Humanism were coming forward. The physical and mental world was in a state of expansion.

In the 1500s and 1600's things began to contract. The first Renaissance ended. Martin Luther and John Calvin sowed the seeds of what would become the Reformation in the creation of their edicts for the church (although technically, Luther was railing against corruption in the Catholic Church, which led to the rise of Protestantism - a more egalitarian interpretation of Christianity. Calvin was instrumental in establishing the tenets of Protestantism, which was one of his main concerns.) This, in turn, lead to the oppression of people like Galileo. The Inquisition raised its ugly head again and persecuted those who enjoyed life, especially women who stood up for themselves.

We have been in this state of contraction for nearly 400 years. Things are starting to rebound as people look for more spiritual rather than religious pursuits. Self Exploration and discovery has become big business. More and more people are appalled by the mistreatment of others and the inequalities in our world. Eco and Humanitarian tourism is everywhere. People want to make a difference and help others.

Let's reclaim the old definition of SENSUALITY. The root of the word is SENSE.

SENSE IS:
- any of the faculties, as sight, hearing, smell, taste, or touch, by which humans and animals perceive stimuli originating from outside or inside the body.
- a feeling or perception produced through the organs of touch, taste, etc., or resulting from a particular sense
- condition of some part of the body: to have a sense of cold
- a faculty or function of the mind analogous to sensation: the moral sense
- any special capacity for perception, estimation, appreciation, etc.: a sense of humour
- to perceive (something) by the senses; become

aware of.
(dictionary.com)

SENSUALITY is all about how we are in the
world, how we interact with it. It has to do with all 5
senses and being fully present in the world with all
those senses. The senses reveal the world to us and
how we respond to our senses is our SENSUALITY.

The book *Extended Massive Orgasm - How you
can give and receive intense sexual pleasure* by
Steve Bodansky, Ph.D. and Vera Bodansky, Ph.D.,
explains the difference between SENSUALITY and
SEXUALITY in this way:
"Sensuality is about giving pleasure to the body
or mind through the senses. The key word here is
pleasure. Sensuality includes all five of our senses:
hearing, seeing, smelling, tasting and touching. It
also includes the sixth sense, which is any use of
conceptual thought to enhance pleasure."
"Sexuality, meanwhile, is the physiological function that pertains to reproduction brought about
by insemination of the female by the male through
penile penetration of the vagina."
I would postulate that SEXUALITY is more
expansive than that clinical definition.

SENSUALITY and SEXUALITY do intertwine.
Since SENSUALITY is how we are in the world - how
we interact and feel - there is no way that SEXUALITY
can't come into it. You can have sex without being
truly SENSUAL. And you can be SENSUAL with no
sex. But both are more fun together!

I feel that SENSUALITY is the culmination of
Self Expression. It's the area seldom explored in
conventional personal development yet it's the

sum of all other pieces put together. Love, anger, fear, sadness, bravery, empathy all roll into one to create our essence, our SENSUALITY. It's the core of who we are and how we are in the world. When you are living your true self in conjunction with your Sensuality, it becomes your AUTHENTIC SENSUALITY.

So do you still not want to be a BAD KITTY? If you're still here, I expect you have a pull to explore it.

Let's look at some BAD KITTIES you may know. You may find one – or more – that you'd like to emulate.

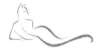

CHAPTER THREE: FAMOUS BAD KITTIES.

There is a perception that to be Sensual you must be really good looking, have a great body and it wouldn't hurt to be rich, either. The truth is that anyone can be Sensual. As we've already discussed, Sensuality is equivalent to Self Expression or authenticity. When you are fully Self Expressed, when you inhabit who you are without reservation, you become Authentically Sensual and your BAD KITTY is released. It doesn't matter what you look like, how much weight you think you need to shed or how much you have in your retirement fund. EVERYONE is Sensual and EVERYONE is a BAD KITTY when they are themselves.

BAD KITTY SCRATCHING POST:

Take a moment and think back to all the people you have known in your life. Whether you ran across them for a moment or have known them since you were a child, see their faces in front of you. Pick out the ones that really stand out; the ones you admired, the ones who inspired you. This is especially true of those you didn't know well. If someone stood out in the crowd at an event or at the mall and you still remember them, put them on the list.

These people that are standing out to you, especially the strangers, are the Authentically Sensual ones. They weren't hiding under false personas. They were letting their light shine and you couldn't help but notice. They are the BAD KITTIES.

THE BAD KITTY'S TAIL:

Those who know me now have a hard time believing that I was once invisible. And yet I was. I went to my 25 year High School reunion recently and most people didn't have a clue who I was or that I was even in their class. I used to be very adept at blending, hiding and not being seen. I wasn't happy with who I was because I didn't know who I was and I didn't want to be found out. Even at 6' tall, I could walk into a room and be completely overlooked.

Now I am never missed. Whenever I go to meet someone for the first time, I describe myself and say, "You can't miss me." I don't even bother getting their description, because I know they'll find me. It helps that I have purple and pink in my hair, but that's certainly not the only factor.

The other day I was walking through a dark parking lot on my way to meet someone. He called out to me. We had never met, but he knew who I was, even in the dark.
It is all about the fact that I radiate myself and my Authentic Sensuality. It's impossible to miss a BAD KITTY!

My facial structure hasn't changed, my body is basically the same, the only thing that has changed is my perception of Self. And that makes all the difference!

I've gone from a woman nobody noticed to one that everyone knows. I've gone from the wallflower to the one who starts the party. I've gone from never being hit on to turning men away. Few changes on the outside, but many changes on the inside and the differences are manifested in all that I do.

CELEBRITY BAD KITTIES:

There are many celebrities that I feel embody Sensuality and live as a BAD KITTY. Some are gorgeous, some are not. What they all have in common is what some would call "Je Ne Sais Quois" - that something special that you can't put your finger on, but you're drawn to them. I know what it is: AUTHENTIC SENSUALITY!

Check out these famous BAD KITTIES and see which ones you identify with.

Please note that bracketed comments after the quotes are my personal comments.

MAE WEST:

My all time favourite and hero – the ultimate BAD KITTY - is Mae West. In the 20's and 30's Sensuality and, especially, Sexuality were even "dirtier" words than they are now. And here was a tiny woman with a knowing smile and a ready wit unafraid to express herself. She had a very sexy edge to her that she displayed in the way she carried herself and in how she spoke. She has the quintessential smoky voice and, with a wink and cock of her eyebrow, she could display more allure than any sex scene in the movies today.

Quotes from Mae West:

- A man can be short and dumpy and getting bald but if he has fire, women will like him. (there's a woman who understands Sensuality!)
- Anything worth doing is worth doing slowly. (Oh, ya!)
- Between two evils, I always pick the one I never tried before.
- Every man I meet wants to protect me. I can't figure out what from.

- He who hesitates is a damned fool.
- I believe that it's better to be looked over than it is to be overlooked. (Say no to invisibility.)
- I never loved another person the way I loved myself. (Double Entendre, love it.)
- I speak two languages, Body and English.
- I used to be Snow White, but I drifted. (I have this one framed on my wall.)
- I'll try anything once, twice if I like it, three times to make sure.
- I'm no model lady. A model's just an imitation of the real thing. (Amen, Sistah!)
- It isn't what I do, but how I do it. It isn't what I say, but how I say it, and how I look when I do it and say it.
- Love thy neighbour - and if he happens to be tall, debonair and devastating, it will be that much easier.
- Marriage is a great institution, but I'm not ready for an institution. (A girl after my own heart)
- Personality is the glitter that sends your little gleam across the footlights and the orchestra pit into that big black space where the audience is.
- Save a boyfriend for a rainy day - and another, in case it doesn't rain.
- When I'm good I'm very, very good, but when I'm bad, I'm better.
- I'm no angel, but I've spread my wings a bit.

BIF NAKED:

I absolutely LOVE Bif Naked. A beautiful Canadian punk rock goddess, she embodies the BAD KITTY. I'm not much for punk in general, but Bif is an exception to so many rules. She is the epitome of contradiction. Incredibly beautiful – she won Miss Naked Vancouver in the 90s and she is also extremely strong in body and mind. She spits on stage, is heavily tattooed and yet is still all girl. She's smart, sexy and artistic and speaks her mind without apology. Her songs are thoughtful, angry and inspiring. Her biggest hit is "I LOVE MYSELF TODAY". It is an anthem of claiming who you are and your power today and every day no matter what has happened to you in the past. Bif is my hero especially now more than ever. She recently won the fight against breast cancer and recorded her new album while going through chemo. Touring with her new shorter hair and the single "Sick", she's more inspiring than ever. The following quotes are poems/rants from Bif's CD inserts.

Quotes from Bif Naked:

- You want an artist's statement? How about EVERYTHING HAPPENS FOR A REASON! or THE MEAN PEOPLE ARE ON THIS EARTH TO TEACH US! or BATHE BECAUSE YOU MUST! or GIVE ME POPCORN OR GIVE ME DEATH! heh heh heh – I feel happy that you are reading this... that is my statement. I feel honoured and privileged that you are reading my words and looking at my cartoons and listening to my songs. Thank you.
- be your own boss. be the boss of your own secret feelings. be yourself. be thankful for your life and your full belly and your shelter. be nice. just be.
- OKAY! A BIG FAT **** OFF IS GOING OUT TO: the insipidity of North America's female body image insistence! AAAAARGH!!! Are we all completely STOOOOPID?! Get REAL, people. Find a higher cause. Go against the grain. Celebrate your uniqueness. Know and

keep your OWN mind – and avoid the delu-
sional. Our society encourages competition
and bitchiness. LET'S RISE ABOVE WHAT
IS EXPECTED OF US AND LOOK AT THE
BIGGER PICTURE: THE PLANET. THE POOR.
THE HOMELESS. THE STARVING. THE
ELDERLY. THE SICK. THE DYING. REALITY.
(Preach it!)
- The opinions I spew are completely my own
  and it is nobody's fault if I say things you
  don't like.
- Um....helooooo!! Get a ****ing hold of yourself!! No complaining!! Are you starving?
  No? Then, let's have a little perspective, shall
  we. See a therapist. Switch to decaf. Lay off
  the pills. Try some stretching. Take five. Have
  a time out. Write it down. Make a painting.
  Have a hot bath. Quit hanging onto the past
  hurts. Forgive all to get over all and get on
  with it! PUH-LEEEZE! Develop some humor.
  Laugh it off. Yuk it up. Don't be mean. Karma
  is instant. There is no coincidence. Live today.
  Try – OK?

MARILYN MONROE:

Then there's Marilyn. I'm speaking of Ms.
Monroe, of course. I love a woman who can be iden-
tified so strongly just by one name. That is truly a
sign of a BAD KITTY. She inspired a generation of
women. She rose out of nothing; from the mousey
Norma Jean to super stardom. A lot of noise is made
about the fact that she was a size 12. In a day when
most actresses starve themselves down to a size 2
no matter their natural figure, this seems unbeliev-
able. She is also sometimes characterized as a
dumb blonde, but she was a smart woman making
her way in a male-dominated world. Unfortunately,

her life ended tragically as she lost her way in the mire of Hollywood, but she started off as a smart and self-assured woman moving through the crazy world of Hollywood and staying true to herself in it all.

Quotes from Marilyn:

- I'm very definitely a woman and I enjoy it. (What's not to enjoy?)
- I don't know who invented high heels, but all women owe him a lot. (Yes, Thank you.)
- I don't mind living in a man's world as long as I can be a woman in it. (Yes, Yes, YES!)
- I don't want to make money. I just want to be wonderful. (This one is on my wall with Mae's)
- People respect you because they feel you've survived hard times and endured, and although you've become famous, you haven't become phony.
- I'm trying to find myself as a person, some-times that's not easy to do. Millions of people live their entire lives without finding them-selves. But it is something I must do.

- That's the trouble, a sex symbol becomes a thing. But if I'm going to be a symbol of some-thing, I'd rather have it sex than some other things we've got symbols of.
- I've often stood silent at a party for hours lis-tening to my movie idols turn into dull and little people. (The Sensual observing the non-Sensual)
- I am invariably late for appointments ... sometimes, as much as two hours. I've tried to change my ways but the things that make me late are too strong, and too pleasing.

MOTHER TERESA:

On a totally different level is Mother Teresa. What? An old shrivelled nun is Sensual? How could a virgin be a BAD KITTY? There are few people in the public eye as completely true to their passion and themselves as this carer of the unclean, the forgotten, those in the greatest need. Her love glowed from every pore. Her touch electrified the masses. She was true to her calling no matter what the obstacle, her mood or the circumstances. She was unstoppable. Now that's a BAD KITTY.

Quotes from Mother Teresa:

- Every time you smile at someone, it is an action of love, a gift to that person, a beautiful thing.
- Being unwanted, unloved, uncared for, forgotten by everybody, I think that is a much greater hunger, a much greater poverty than the person who has nothing to eat.
- Do not think that love, in order to be genuine, has to be extraordinary. What we need is to love without getting tired.
- I have found the paradox, that if you love until it hurts, there can be no more hurt, only more love.
- I know God will not give me anything I can't handle. I just wish that He didn't trust me so much. (Yes, she was human.)
- It is not the magnitude of our actions but the amount of love that is put into them that matters.
- Kind words can be short and easy to speak, but their echoes are truly endless.
- We ourselves feel that what we are doing is just a drop in the ocean. But the ocean would

be less because of that missing drop.

ELLEN DEGENERES:

Sensuality is Fun and no one embodies that better than
Ellen Degeneres. She is an infectious personality. She loves to dance. She dresses in what makes her feel comfortable and suits her personality. She laughs and makes everyone around her join in. Once she came out many years ago, her impact changed. Up until then she was just another funny woman. After she was honest about her sexuality, and therefore true to her Sensuality, she became a force to bc reckoned with because she was no longer hiding a very key part of who she is. She became a BAD KITTY to watch.

Quotes from Ellen:

For me, it's that I contributed,...that I'm on this planet doing some goog and making people happy. That's to me the most important thing, that my hour of television is positive and upbeat and an antidote for all the negative stuff going on in life.

I gotta work out. I keep saying that all the time, I keep saying I gotta start working out. It's been about two months since I've worked out. And I just don't have the time. Which uh...is odd. Because I have the time to go out to dinner. And uh...and waqtch tv. And get a bone density test. And uh... try to figure out what my phone number spells in words.

I don't understand the sizes anymore. There's a size zero, which I didn't even know that they had. It must stand for: 'Ohhh my God, you're thin.'

Sometimes you can't see yourself clearly until you see yourself through the eyes of others.

Sometimes when I'm driving I get so angry at inconsiderate drivers that I want to scream at them. But then I remember how insignificant that is, and I thank God that I have a car and my health and gas. That was phrased wrong - normally you wouldn't say, thank God I have gas.

You have funny faces and words, you can't just have words. It is a powerful thing, and I think that's why it's hard for people to imagine that women can do that, be that powerful.

OPRAH:

Another powerful force is Oprah. This BAD KITTY could rule the world. She is not only the most powerful, and richest, black woman in the world, but quite possibly the most powerful - and certainly best known - woman in the world, period. She has had a passion and drive that has never waned. Her Sensuality shows through in her willingness to share, to be open, to reveal her struggles. Her willingness allows others to do the same. Her passion to help has opened doors and hearts for multitudes.

Quotes from Oprah:

- As you become more clear about who you really are, you'll be better able to decide what is best for you - the first time around.
- Be thankful for what you have; you'll end up having more. If you concentrate on what you don't have, you will never, ever have enough. (What you focus on expands.)
- Breathe. Let go. And remind yourself that this very moment is the only one you know you have for sure.
- Doing the best at this moment puts you in the best place for the next moment.
- I am a woman in process. I'm just trying like

everybody else. I try to take every conflict, every experience, and learn from it. Life is never dull.

- I don't think you ever stop giving. I really don't. I think it's an on-going process. And it's not just about being able to write a check. It's being able to touch somebody's life.
- I still have my feet on the ground, I just wear better shoes. (Great shoes are vital.)
- Real integrity is doing the right thing, knowing that nobody's going to know whether you did it or not.
- I feel that luck is preparation meeting opportunity.
- We can't become what we need by remaining what we are. (We are either growing or dying, which one are you?)

GILDA RADNER:

Gilda Radner was a funny, smart and fearless woman. She fought anorexia and bulimia as a youth. She went on to be one of the most famous women on Saturday Night Live. She inspired many with her fight against ovarian cancer which eventually took her light from us in 1989. Her inspiration and love led her husband Gene Wilder and other friends to create the Gilda Club. It was Gilda's wish that a place be established where people of all ages diagnosed with cancer could come together and support one another. The centers are non- medical and homey including an art center, exercise facility, game rooms, and a children's room called Noogieland, so named for "noogies", one of Gilda's comedic actions. Gilda's Club is now North America-wide, with new centers opening up all over the United States and Canada. She is greatly missed by many, including me. I had the opportunity to perform one of her

Roseanne Roseannadanna bits and feel especially connected to Gilda's indomitable spirit.

Quotes from Gilda:

- While we have the gift of life, it seems to me the only tragedy is to allow part of us to die - whether it is our spirit, our creativity or our glorious uniqueness.
- Life is about not knowing, having to change, taking the moment and making the best of it, without knowing what's going to happen next.
- I'd much rather be a woman than a man. Women can cry, they can wear cute clothes, and they're the first to be rescued off sinking ships.
- I base my fashion sense on what doesn't itch.
- Dreams are like paper, they tear so easily.
- I can always be distracted by love, but eventually I get horny for my creativity.
- I wanted a perfect ending. Now I've learned, the hard way, that some poems don't rhyme, and some stories don't have a clear beginning, middle and end.

JAMIE LEE CURTIS:

In 2002 actress and author Jamie Lee Curtis did an amazingly brave and inspiring BAD KITTY thing. She called *More* magazine and proposed they do a photo shoot of her without makeup or stylists. The idea was to show women the world over that even the stars look like the rest of us. As proof, she also did a photo shoot with 13 stylists and 3 hours work as a contrast. She put female beauty as shown in popular culture into perspective. Her truth and bravery is Sensual.

Quotes from Jamie Lee:

- I think happiness comes from self-accept-ance. We all try different things, and we find some comfortable sense of who we are. We look at our parents and learn and grow and move on. We change.
- I talk too much. (Sensual women know them-selves and own it.)
- I think I felt that I was very well known for my figure and needed to keep that up for my work. And I regret all of it. I felt fraudulent and very shameful.
- I think my capacity to change has given me tremendous happiness, because who I am today I am completely content to be.
- I thought, while they're up and firm, why not shoot them once or twice.
- I was doing a children's book on self-esteem, and I really felt like I wanted to shed the shame I'd been feeling –
    and maybe make it easier for women my age who had probably felt bad about them-selves.
- The more I like me, the less I want to pretend to be other people. (That's the BAD KITTY key.)

KIM CATTRALL:

A modern melding of Marilyn and Mae West is Kim Cattrall. She embodies both Sensuality and Sexuality fully. In her 50's, she is amazing and free in who she is. As the oldest cast member of Sex and the City, she was the one most willing to do nude scenes. She isn't swayed by the youth culture. She knows she is vital in all areas of her life at her age, and possibly even more so. We can all be a BAD KITTY at any age.

Quotes from Kim:

- Art is an expression of who you are. Parts that I play are my sculptures.
- I sort of have a love affair with my work. Many of us work far too hard and we don't put enough value in the epicurean, sensual part of life. (Overworked and overwhelmed – let's just say NO!)
- I'm a trisexual. I'll try anything once. (Love it, my new motto.)
- I've always thought that less was a lot more.
- I'm certainly not a prude.
- Really rejoice in being yourself. Have your own drumbeat. (Please, everyone.)
- That's what life is - you follow where your heart leads you - at least I do.

AUDREY HEPBURN:

Audrey Hepburn is an icon of class. Everything about her is feline, so BAD KITTY. From her baby doll youth to the poise in her senior years, Audrey was inspiring. Her carriage was always composed. She had strong beliefs that she quietly and passionately pursued. She didn't push herself on others; she let her actions speak for themselves. She was beautiful, but her true beauty was in her love of children and her support of groups like UNICEF and her own charity, The Audrey Hepburn Children's Fund. Audrey was innately Sensual in her expression and in her love of life and others.

Quotes from Audrey:

- For beautiful eyes, look for the good in others; for beautiful lips, speak only words of kindness; and for poise, walk with the knowledge that you are never alone. (Thank you, so beautifully put.)

- I love people who make me laugh. I honestly think it's the thing I like most, to laugh. It cures a multitude of ills. It's probably the most important thing in a person.
- I never think of myself as an icon. What is in other people's minds is not in my mind. I just do my thing.
- I was asked to act when I couldn't act. I was asked to sing 'Funny Face' when I couldn't sing, and dance with Fred Astaire when I couldn't dance - and do all kinds of things I wasn't prepared for. Then I tried like mad to cope with it. (BAD KITTIES are willing to rise to challenges.)
- I was born with an enormous need for affection, and a terrible need to give it.
- People, even more than things, have to be restored, renewed, revived, reclaimed, and redeemed; never throw out anyone.
- Remember, if you ever need a helping hand, it's at the end of your arm, as you get older, remember you have another hand: The first is to help yourself, the second is to help others.

QUEEN LATIFAH:

When a Big Beautiful Woman carries herself with pride and refuses to give in to the conventional standards of beauty pushed on us by the film and fashion industry, I am thrilled and inspired. Queen Latifah is one such BBBK – a Big Beautiful BAD KITTY. Even though I'm sure she has been constantly bombarded by publicists and producers telling her to lose weight, she keeps her glorious curves. She has such an obvious lust for life, a wonderful sense of humour and is gorgeous on her terms. She exudes Sensuality from her essence.

Quotes from Queen Latifah:

- I made decisions that I regret, and I took them as learning experiences ... I'm human, not perfect, like anybody else.
- I was taught from a young age that many people would treat me as a second-class citizen because I was African-American and because I was female. (And she rose to the top anyway – love ya baby!)
- I think the reason I am here is to inspire African-American women who are rappers, full-figured women to know that they can do it too. (And we non-rapping women in general as well.)
- There are times you can't really see or even feel how sweet life can be. Hopefully its mountains will be higher than its valleys are deep. I know things that are broken can be fixed. Take the punch if you have to, hit the canvas and then get up again. Life is worth it.
- I really don't know how to be anyone else, and whenever I try to be anyone else, I fail miserably.

Are you inspired yet? Do you see parts of yourself in these women? Did some of the quotes speak to you? Do you see what makes them BAD KITTIES? Did you notice that each BAD KITTY is unique?

I put this together and have read through it many times. Even now some of the quotes will really speak to me. Sometimes they are the same ones as previously, other times something new will pop out. I am continually inspired to be my best by these women.

BAD KITTY SCRATCHING POST:

Take another moment to go though the quotes. Check off or highlight the ones that stand out to you and speak to your inner BAD KITTY. Take sticky notes or index cards and write them out. Post them on your mirror, your desk, your fridge. Put them up where you can be constantly reminded of their inspiration.

I have one of Mae's and Marilyn's quotes framed in my bedroom with their pictures. I love the quotes themselves, and having them there reminds me of the fabulous women to which they are attributed. Just knowing they are there smiling at me, facing my bed every morning and night gives me a lift.

BAD KITTY SCRATCHING POST:

Think back on those people who stood out to you in your life that you thought about at the beginning of this chapter. Visualize them. Write down their names, or descriptions if they are stand out strangers. Make a list of what it is about them that you admire. Why are they a BAD KITTY? It could simply be the great haircut and purse of that woman in the Safeway line. It could be a long list of the wonderful things a friend has done for you or the qualities of that special someone.

Celebrate these people in your life. Let as many as you can know what you appreciate about them. Let them know that you love how they express themselves and contribute to your life in a positive way. They will want to know why you call them a BAD KITTY!

The next time you see a stranger who stands out, go up to them and tell them what you see. "Oh,

I love your jacket." "I couldn't help but notice you, you carry yourself so confidently." "Where did you get those shoes?" Make someone's day by acknowledging them. It will lift your spirits as well when you get a big smile and Thank You.

Keep your eyes open for those who embody AUTHENTIC SENSUALITY and THE BAD KITTY. You may be surprised where they come from. Look for those who are exuding their BEAUTY by being THEMSELVES.

Happy BAD KITTY hunting!

CHAPTER FOUR: HERE KITTY, KITTY, KITTY

I hope you were inspired by the famous BAD KITTIES in the previous chapter. There are so many more. It would be easy to do a whole book just on them and maybe I will at some point. For now, I'm sure that the ones I shared gave you a good over-view of what's possible and how many different Kitties there are out there. I hope you found one like yourself, or the self you can see buried deep inside.

I have observed many women losing or squelch-ing their AUTHENTIC SENSUALITY. They lose their BAD KITTY selves in so many ways. It is sad to see that light go out. To see it struggling to come back and being pushed down over and over again. Thankfully our AUTHENTIC SENSUALITY is part and parcel of who we are and it will return given the opportunity. But how does it disappear in the first place?

THE BAD KITTY'S TAIL:

There are so many stories I could tell here and some of the stories I have already shared show examples of how my own self and AUTHENTIC SENSUALITY were pushed down. Spoiler alert, this is one of the most traumatic.

My mother remarried when I was 12. He was a Viet Nam vet and an alcoholic. He was a mission-ary kid and had expectations of himself to save the world in between his bouts of alcoholism and even while drunk in the bar. He had high standards for the family and set a lot of strict rules, such as no more than 2 hours of TV per week. He put the TV in a cupboard in the basement at one point. We were all expected to attend church and Sunday School each week, as well as Bible studies and church youth activities. We had family Bible study time, said grace at each meal and could only listen to "Christian" music.

Now, please hear me, none of this is inherently wrong. I am thankful in many ways that I grew up in this way as it kept me out of trouble. I didn't drink, do drugs or have sex in high school. Even to this day, I've never done drugs or been drunk. My friends were all "good" kids who wanted to make a difference in the world and stay pure.

The trouble came on the day that he came into my room in the middle of the night. I was in grade 10. I was a late bloomer and didn't hit puberty until 16. I was "safe". I had very low self esteem. My younger sister "blossomed" before I did. She was the "pretty" one. She had the interest of boys. I was the invisible one.

Over a thankfully short period of time, I was molested by my step father. There's no need to go into the details. Considering that 42% of women report being abused as a child, I'm sure everyone reading this has either been there or knows some-one who has.

Most of the actual physical activity has been compartmentalized and I remember very little of it. I do, however, remember vividly one comment that was made. In his drunken voice he whispered, "I chose you because you're sexier than your sister, but she shows it."

It was like he was trying to give me a positive message as he was putting his hands where they didn't belong. Instead, the "sexiness" (as he put it), my SENSUALITY and sense of self (as I see it), went deeper inside and hid. If that part of me was inviting this sort of attention when it wasn't fully realized, what would it do if I let it loose! I put it away to keep myself safe.

I'm surprised at how difficult that section was to write. There are some things, no matter how much work is done around them or how far I think I'm removed from it, that can still bring up emotions. It is more about the time lost, the self lost during that long period than about the event itself. Everything we experience makes us who we are. On the positive side, I am a more caring person, more empathetic and able to see how traumatic events affect people. It has added to my passion to help women bring out their AUTHENTIC SENSUALITY in healthy ways and to help them see that it is not dangerous, scary or wrong, but rather fun, real and honest.

THE BAD KITTY'S TAIL:

I mentioned in Chapter 1 that I had been married. Technically, we were together for 8 years. I say technically because in the 7th year, he went overseas. No, he wasn't in the military. He was too skinny and they wouldn't take him! He went to Korea to teach English.

Originally, I was to join him there; but he didn't make as much money as he was expecting and it never did happen. Our communication was limited to some online chatting, letters and rare phone calls.

He had a one year contract. At the 9 month mark he came home for a visit. I was directing a play for the youth at our church and he showed up in the middle of rehearsal. I was over the moon! I ran to him and smiled so wide my face hurt. The youth were almost as happy to see him, as he used to run their group. He got mobbed.

We had a great few days catching up, having plenty of sex and once again feeling connected. It wasn't until his last night in town that I found out the real reason for his visit.

We were out for pizza at a full restaurant in the University area. About half way through the meal he said, "I need to tell you why I came back." Immediately, my mind started to reel. What reason could there be? He needed to see me, he needed a break. What else could there possibly be? This can't be good. "I'm not sure I want to be married anymore."

The rest of the conversation is a blur. I know I cried a lot. I know I tried to keep it quiet so as not to make a scene. I know that I wanted to understand. One answer he kept giving was "I don't know." Now I wouldn't accept that answer, but then I did. One question I posed was, "Now what?" The stock "I don't know" answer was given. I had to step up. My solution was that he had 3 months left on his contract so he had until then to decide what he wanted.

In that 3 month period, I knew what was going to happen. I was mentally preparing myself. He wasn't good at making difficult decisions, so I knew it would come down to me. I began, subconsciously, to be single again.

When the year ended he still "didn't know" what he wanted, so I said that it was over. We had no property or children, so we split up our stuff that was in storage and I filed a do it yourself divorce. He went back to Korea.

I felt like a failure. I was a good church girl. Marriage is supposed to be forever. There must be something wrong with me. I must be a bad wife, an undesirable woman, a waste of time and energy, someone disposable. For a long time I couldn't stand to be alone. I had to have the affirmation from a man that I was OK.

On the positive side, I found I could make the tough choices and I didn't have to follow the expectations of others. I could go through something that cut me to my core and come out stronger and more assured on the other side. I was released to explore me and what I wanted in life rather than what "we" wanted – or, in our case, what HE wanted. I met people I never would have met if we were together and had opportunities I would have missed out on. I started on a path that brought me here. I am thankful for him not wanting to be married anymore! I can't begin to imagine how miserable we would both be if we were still together.

BAD KITTY SCRATCHING POST:

I promise, soon we will be doing some activities with more action. Right now, we still need to be in reflection. We'll get there!

Sit quietly with your notebook and pen beside you. Close your eyes and look back. Are there events in your life that made you close down? It can be something obviously traumatic or something much smaller. It can be rejection by someone you loved. It can be being told that you were ugly or stupid. It can be a friend asking "why did you do *that?*" in that sharp, sarcastic way that can cut to the quick.

Write out this story – or stories – in as much detail as you can remember. What was going on around you? What sights, sounds and smells do you recall? What feelings were you having? What sensations did you have in your body? What did you think about yourself and how did it affect you?

Once finished, read the story out loud. Read it with the intention of releasing the thoughts and feelings related to it. If willing, read it to someone else so that you can give it away and have someone else witness your process.

Now go back to your notebook and write down what you learned from this event. What positive effects has it had? How did it help you in your life? What gifts have you been given as a result of the pain?

Read this out loud and celebrate. Read it in a happy, excited voice. Throw in some WooHoos or Yippeees. Stand up as you read. Use your arms and body to emphasize your excitement. When you are done reading, look up and say Thank you!

Notice the changes in your body. Notice the changes in your feelings. Remember that everything has something good in behind it, no matter what pain is felt in the moment. Celebrate every moment!

BIRTH OF STANDARDS:

We all grow up with Standards. Standards are the mores of behaviour that we are taught as we grow. They are expressed in direct and subliminal ways. They get into our heads and we begin to think they are true, right and good for us. Sometimes this is true, sometimes it's not. Often we spend many years thinking something is wrong with us because we fight to fit ourselves into the standards set for us by others.

Where do these standards come from? They usually come from sources of authority – parents, teachers, religious leaders, caregivers, coaches, club leaders, camp counsellors, bus drivers, police, crossing guards, and many more. Wow, when you start thinking about it, we have a lot of authority figures telling us what to do! They can also come from people on our level; friends and peers. It's no wonder we grow up pulled in so many directions and sometimes forget who we are!

THE BAD KITTY'S TAIL:

Before I tell this story, let me clarify that I love my mom. We are a lot alike so sometimes we clash. I have always admired her. She has been through a lot of struggles with divorce, tight finances, single momhood and an alcoholic first and second husband. She makes the best of situations and finds ways to make things work. I know that she has done her best in everything with what she knew and I can't fault her for doing her best.

Like a pebble in a pond everything we do affects those around us. If the universe was a lake there would be millions of little round ripples all overlapping and intersecting each other. We can't help but affect each other's lives in ways that are visible and invisible.

I grew up with an expectation, a standard. I was the strong one. My sister was the pretty one. My mom's favourite story to tell about me was when I was 3 I decided I wanted my dresser moved. It was my nap time and I guess it was bothering me somehow. I got up and moved it; a 5 drawer high boy full of clothes. I moved it across the room by myself.

I felt that if I wasn't exhibiting strength, then I wouldn't be loved. I refused to cry in front of others. When I did I was made fun of. My sister and mom would cry openly at a movie without recriminations. If I cried – or was seen crying – it was pointed out with a sneer. As a result, I would do everything I could to hold it in until I could let it out without being observed.

I developed such a hard shell that my sister called me Spock. If there was anything that showed weakness, I ran from it. If I wasn't good at something that was a sign of weakness, so I would just stay away from it. I'm sure I lost out on many interesting opportunities that would have come if I had just worked on things I wasn't immediately good at a little more.

I would sometimes get a bullying attitude because if people didn't do what I wanted, then that was weak. I always had to be in control in every situation. Any feeling of a lack of control would send me into a rage. I had temper tantrums until I was 12 because that was the only way I knew how to get that rage out when something went against what I wanted. It was my way of showing strength in weakness. Eventually I figured out it wasn't all that effective!

The need for control created so many ripple effects, I'm still discovering them. It created a discomfort in my own skin. The need to be strong and live up to the expectations I felt were being put on me made me into someone I didn't like very much.

THE MOMENT OF DISCOVERY:

Many years down the road, I took a personality test called True Colors. It breaks down personalities into four colors.

Orange represents energy, action, consuming physiological potency, power, and strength. Orange is the expression of vital force, of nervous and glandular activity. Thus, it has the meaning of desire and all forms of appetite and craving. Those with Orange as a Primary Color feel the will to achieve results, to win, to be successful. They desire all things that offer intense living and full experience. Orange generates an impulse toward active doing: sport, struggle, competition and enterprising productivity. It stimulates enthusiasm and creativity. Orange means vitality with endurance. In temporal terms, Orange is the present.

Gold is the body's natural perceptions. It represents a need to be responsible, to fulfill duties and obligations, to organize and structure our life and that of others. Those with Gold as a Primary Color value being practical and sensible; they believe that people should earn their way in life through work and service to others. Gold reflects a need to belong through carrying a share of the load in all areas of living. It represents stability, maintenance of the culture and the organization, efficiency, planning and dependability. It embraces the concepts of home and family with fierce loyalty and faithfulness.

Green expresses itself psychologically as human will in operation: as persistence and determination. Green is an expression of firmness and consistency. Its strength can lead to a resistance to change if it is not proven that the change will work or is warranted. Those with Green as a Primary Color value their intellect and capabilities above all else. Comfort in these areas creates a sense of personal security and self-esteem. Green characteristics seek to increase the certainty of their own values through being assertive and requiring differences from others in intellectual areas. They are rarely settled in their countenance, since they depend upon information rather than feelings to create a sense of well-being. Green expresses the grounding of theory and data in its practical applications and creative constructs.

Blue represents calm. Contemplation of this color pacifies the central nervous system. It creates physiological tranquility and psychological content- ment. Those with Blue as a Primary Color value balance and harmony. They prefer lives free from tension... settled, united, and secure. Blue rep- resents loyalty and a sense of belonging, and yet, when friends are involved, a vulnerability. Blue cor- responds to depth in feeling and a relaxed sensitiv- ity. It is characterized by empathy, aesthetic experi- ences, and reflective awareness. Blue is the color of inspiration, sincerity and spirituality. Blue is often the chosen color by conservative people. Using Blue to relax will encourage feelings of communication and peace.

From www.truecolors.org
In a nutshell, Orange is the Actor, the free spirit. Gold is the organizer. Green is the analyzer. Blue is the People Person.

All the colors have their place in the world. They are all wonderful and necessary. Every person is a combination of all, but has a primary one that rules the way they proceed through life.

When I first took the test, I came out as primarily Gold. It made me annoyed. I didn't like being Gold. But it is how I had lived my life for so long that I didn't know any other way to be.

I took the test again in a larger group a year later. We split the room into the colors. I knew a lot of people in the room. Many of them came up to me afterwards and said, "What were you doing in the Gold group, you're so Orange!" I got defensive. I get that way when I'm in the Gold place.

It wasn't until a few years later that I really understood what was going on. It's not that my natural color is Gold, it's that I lived in that place of control and the overdeveloped sense of being responsible for everything that I THOUGHT I was Gold. The fact that I felt so out of sorts when I was living in that energy was one sign that it was imposed on me rather than being my true expression.

It wasn't until I started living Orange that I really started to love my life. Deep down I am very competitive. I love a challenge! I love trying new things and exploring new ideas. Now that I don't feel the need to be right and perfect all the time I can enjoy who I really am. I am having so much fun living Orange! I can go into the Gold when I need some efficiency and structure and I can own and enjoy my Orange self that I covered over for so many years.

Standards aren't inherently bad. They aren't inherently good. They just are. The thing is, they belong to someone else. They have been passed down from generation to generation and we come to passively accept them as true. They may have been true and useful when they were created hundreds of years ago, but are they still? Just because they're right for someone else, does that mean they're right for you?

THE BAD KITTY'S TAIL:

I grew up in a Christian home. After my parents divorced my mom became a Christian and my sister and I followed. We went to church and Sunday School almost every week. I was involved in drama productions, youth groups, choirs and formed a trio in high school. My world revolved around what I was told by the church.

I wanted to be a missionary. As I mentioned earlier, when I found out my ex husband wanted to be a youth pastor, I felt I'd hit the jackpot.

Problem was I was never fully comfortable with the restrictions put on me by the traditional church. I always felt I was in a straight jacket. I began to think that this was how it was supposed to be. I wanted to please God and my mom and the pastors and be a good girl so I'd just have to suck it up. I was rigid and judgemental. I looked down at anyone who wasn't following the Word and couldn't understand why.

After my divorce, I didn't go to church for awhile. I didn't go back to the one that my ex and I attended. I knew there would be sideways glances and judgements that I didn't want to deal with. I was a leader and now I was divorced. That was bad and wrong.

Eventually I started going to a new church when I was living in a new city. I had been attending several weeks when they had a sharing time about a big revival retreat that had recently occurred. I listened to several people get up and talk about how much they learned about being open and inviting and reaching out to the community.

I couldn't handle it and went to the mike. "I didn't

go to the retreat," I said, "I have been coming to this church for several weeks. In that time not one person has greeted me, talked to me or in any way made me feel welcome. Everything you're saying is great and I hope you do it. But take a look at what's going on here first. How do you treat the people who have already come to you? I am divorced and was afraid to come back to church because of how I saw my mother treated as a second class citizen after her divorce by the people in her church. Look at yourselves – will new people feel welcome here? From my experience the answer is no."

I stayed for the rest of the service. No one approached me afterwards. I never went back.

I'm not saying that church or church people are bad. I'm saying it did not work for me and it took a dramatic event for me to really get that. I felt liberated by releasing those standards. Some of them work for me still, but as a whole, I had to release them and take back what was right for me. Honesty, treating others well, respecting people no matter their situation, generosity, forgiveness and love are all great standards. The culture of the church was what wasn't working.

BAD KITTY SCRATCHING POST:

Have you ever stood up for yourself? Have you made a shift in your life that changed your direction in a way that was unexpected and exciting?

Record this moment in as much detail as you can. Write down what happened; who was there, where was it, what sensations did you have. What was the result? How are things different for you now?

Read this story aloud, preferably with an audience of at least one. When done, celebrate. Do high fives and cheer. Put on some music and dance. Treat yourself to something you've been putting off. You deserve it. You are in control of your life!

Are there times in your life that you wish you would have said or done something? Is there something now that you need to deal with? Is there something you've been putting off because you're afraid of what might happen on the other side? Is there a job you need to leave? A relationship you need to end? A friend you need to tell the truth? A communication that's gone unresolved? A family member with whom you need to set boundaries?

Write out the details of this situation or situations. Why are you stopping yourself from dealing with it? If, or rather when, you take care of it, what will change? What positive outcomes do you see happening? Go into the future by a few years. How will your life be different? How will you be different?

Feel the energy of this positive outcome wash over you. See yourself in this new light.

Now set a commitment as to when and how you are going to deal with this. You know it must be done; putting it off only makes it harder. If possible, set the intention for completion less than 3 days in advance. Just do it, baby! You know you wanna.

In a nutshell, we lose our SENSUALITY by letting the expectations of others and the sad, traumatic or less than perfect events in our lives close us off.

Look at a child. When they are young, everything is possible, nothing is off limits. They cry unabashedly when they're sad. They scream with pleasure.

There is nothing as pure as the laughter of a child. They are hungry when they're hungry and don't live by a schedule. They look directly in your eyes without agenda. Their only expectation is that you return their love and meet their needs.

THE BAD KITTY'S TAIL:

I have no children. I love children. It occurred to me recently that one reason I didn't want any of my own is because I don't want to be responsible for breaking them! I have observed my nieces and nephews and friend's kids grow up. I've seen them go from wide open infants and toddlers to becoming increasingly closed down and guarded as they grow. I couldn't handle knowing that something I did as a flawed human contributed to that!

Currently, my favourite person in the world is my Grand Niece, Emily. How can you not love someone who comes barrelling to the door calling your name when you walk in? She will hold my face and look right in my eyes. She gives kisses and hugs freely. She says exactly what she wants in every moment. Her emotions change on a dime. She loves to explore, to play, and to just be! I love being around that energy. It enlivens me.

All my nieces and nephews were in this place at one time. I don't love them any less now that they're grown, but being around a 3 year old energy cannot be matched by anything else in terms of purity.

A few years ago my friend Sabrina's son, Alexander, was 3. He loved me. It was hard to visit with his mom because he wanted all my attention. He, like most kids, loved to play with me. I don't put my agenda on games and kids love that. They get to run the show. He wanted all my attention and often asked his mom if I could babysit.

One day I was in a rocky place as I had just been dumped. I was feeling a sorry for myself, confused and broken. I went to Sabrina's house and Alexander ran to the door screaming my name to give me a big hug. Sabrina said, "Anytime you're having man trouble, just come over here."

Unfortunately, now that he is older, I don't get the same enthusiastic welcome from Alex and I understand that,

unfortunately, that's part of growing up. What I wonder is, does it have to be?

A person's true self is reflected in those early years. We haven't yet learned to adjust ourselves to what we think others expect of us. We haven't yet been told by others what's "right" or "acceptable". Yes, there are some rules of society we have to live by so there isn't complete anarchy. And within those rules there is a lot of room to allow the individual. It's our true selves that make life interesting. It's our true selves that make us happy. It's our true selves that are SENSUAL.

If we all lived as we are rather than by the rules imposed by outside sources, there would be no war, no crime, no hate. If only, somehow, we could learn to open our hearts and see how beautiful everyone is no matter their religion, culture or sexual orientation. If only we could see that we are all, at the core, the same!

We all have the same struggles, the same issues, the same fears, the same joys. We are more alike than we like to let on. It's because we stay closed off that we never know these things. If we knew that that weird guy on the corner grew up in the same neighbourhood, went to the same school and loved the same teacher, we would look at him differently. If only we knew that the woman who seems so full of herself is over-compensating for a fear of intimacy, we would have more patience. If we knew that the boss who makes such crazy demands was abused as a child we would look at the source of those expectations differently.

A BAD KITTY has come to terms with the expectations forced on her by others and has come back to her true, full and expressive AUTHENTIC SENSUALITY. She understands that others may not be there yet. She understands that it is a journey and is willing to do what it takes to shed the habits, standards and behaviours that aren't working.

It's time to go there. Are you brave enough to go on? I thought so.

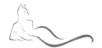

CHAPTER FIVE:

MAKING THE BAD KITTY PURRRRRRR

THE BAD KITTY'S TAIL:

In 2002 I took a course called _The Mastery of Self Expression_. This is the most interactive and powerful weekend I'd ever had before and have had since. It was created in the 70's by Dan Fauci – a producer and director in New York – who saw that actors were losing their passion for their craft.

Having been an actor, or aspiring to be, I know how easily that can happen. When I was in the "I can't sell" part of my life, one reason I gave was not being able to handle rejection. Ironically, that's exactly what you get most of the time as an actor. And they're not rejecting a product, they're rejecting you! You're too tall, too short, too pretty, not pretty enough, too skinny, too fat, too white, too dark, too old, too young, too experienced, not the right experience. It goes on and on and it's all about YOU! No wonder actors get discouraged.

As Dan Fauci developed the workshop, he realized that people in general had lost their passion. They had lost their sense of self. They were stuck in a box and didn't know how to get out. They were living by other people's standards and suffocating. He opened the workshop up to the general public and thousands of people around the world thank him for doing so.

I'm one of those thousands. I had taken quite a lot of personal development when I discovered *The Mastery*. I was working with *Peak Potentials* and had done 7 courses over about 3 years. I am very grateful to Peaks and T. Harv Eker for starting me on a growth path.

Through Peaks, I was introduced to *The Mastery*. My life was different from Peaks, but it wasn't until I did *The Mastery* that things gelled and changes came fast and furious. The life I dreamed about in exercises and visualizations was now coming true!

Over the years of working with *The Mastery* as an assistant and a facilitator, I've had a lot of my blocks come clear and have faced the demons of my own misconceptions. The first I became aware of was my inability, and unwillingness, to ask for help. Having acted so self sufficiently for so long, it was something completely foreign to me. Not only did I have a habit of just doing things, but I also expected that even if I asked for it, I wouldn't get the help I needed in the way I expected it. For the latter, I came to understand that I wasn't being clear in my requests. People wanted to help - but if I didn't give those exact requests, they would interpret the situation, and my needs, as they saw it and then I would be frustrated.

That one shift created a chain reaction that has continued to blossom and expand.

- I've come from being in low wage service industry jobs to having my own successful business.
- I've come from barely scraping by every month with a used car and renting to leasing

new cars, buying a house and having many fabulous shoes.

- I've come from little Miss Invisible to Ms. Can't Be Missed.
- I've come from feeling that my ideas were shallow and unworthy to being called an inspiration.
- I've come from dreaming about being an author to accomplishing it.
- I've come from dreaming about being onstage to having opportunities to speak in front of large groups.
- I've come from hating myself to loving myself.

Do any of those befores resonate with you?

Maybe you are already at some of the afters and want more.

HABITS:

We all have habits. They range from the order we do tasks in our morning routine to how we react in certain situations. Most habits are unconscious. We do them so automatically that we don't even think about it until something throws a wrench into that routine.

I live alone, so usually my routines are uninterrupted. When I have someone else at my house I feel out of sorts. All of a sudden someone's in my bathroom when I need it. The person who just had a shower didn't put the bathmat back on the side of the tub. The guest who helped with the dishes didn't put the ladle back in the right spot and now I can't find it. I tend to do a fair bit of lost ambling about when I have others visiting. It takes awhile to acclimatize to other people's habits.

Many of our habits are innocuous. If we do them
- or don't - it's not the end of the world. If I brush
my teeth before or after I wash my face, it makes no
difference. If I don't make my bed this morning, it's
not going to hurt anyone.

Some habits have positive results; parking a
little further from the mall so you get a little exercise, repeating a person's name when you meet
them so you remember it, washing your hands.

Sometimes we do things so unconsciously we
don't even realize that they're not serving us, that
they're actually creating tension or disharmony in
our lives. From being consistently late to not really
listening to others to not following through on promises made – we create negative results around us.

It's easy to make excuses like "well, I tried my
best" or "that's just the way I am" or "it isn't all
that important." The fact is that every action we do
is very important. Everything we do creates ripples
around us. Positive or negative, those ripples are
going out into the world. What kind do you want to
create?

Think for a moment. For example, if you are
someone who makes promises or commitments
without thought, how do you feel when someone
says they are going to call you or help you out and
they don't follow through? The first time, you might
forgive them. The second time get annoyed, the
third time angry and the fourth time you'll think
twice before asking again. Some people will cut off
sooner, some later, but the result is eventually the
same – distrust, disappointment and a damaged
relationship. Unless that is what you want around
you, it's time to look at your habits.

BAD KITTY SCRATCHING POST:

There is an old axiom called "Act as If." This is an acting exercise as well as a way to live your life. It's the old "Fake it till you Make it." When we want to change our behaviour, we need to "act as if" we are already what/who/how we want to be.

If you are chronically late, rather than always talking about and accepting that you're always late, make a decision not to be late for a week. Make the adjustments in your schedule and mind set. If you have kids, you know that they will take some time to get ready, so make allowances for that. If you're travelling at rush hour, know that you will need to leave earlier. If you need gas or to stop and pick up milk, be sure to factor that in. Make a decision to actually be early and see how it feels.

If you are shy in a group, make a decision to start a conversation with at least 2 people at the next group activity you go to. If you are so shy that you shy away (pun intended) from group events, then make a decision to go anyway! Really push yourself and go to something at least once a week for a month and start conversations every time. Yes, it will be hard and uncomfortable and do it anyway.

If you hate to ask for help, make a decision to ask for help once a day, even if it's something you can easily do. Get the bag boy to carry your groceries. Ask your husband to cook supper once this week. Ask a stranger to help you get a box off a high shelf in the store. There are many opportunities every day to ask for help. When you start to be open to it, you will notice that people offer help frequently and we often say, "No, that's ok". It's time to say, "Yes, thank you so much!" Remember to say thank you!

Take a moment to think of one habit or behaviour you would really like to change in your life; something that really isn't working for you. Something you do more out of habit than choice. Something that makes you or others around you nuts.

Make a conscious choice to do something different for at least a week. Notice that it gets easier each time you do it. If you continue it for a month, eventually you won't even notice how easy it's become. The habit will have changed. It takes 21 days to develop a new habit. Your sensibility will have changed. Your sense of self will have changed in a positive way.

Isn't that worth a little discomfort at the start? For me it sure was!

FILTERS:

One crazy making thing we as humans do is to make a decision that this is how it is, "This is me" and shrug our shoulders as if it can't be any different. "If you don't like me, then too bad - this is me." This is self defeating. It's a way of ignoring things that aren't working and pretending it doesn't matter.

The question is, is it really you? Or is it something you've just gotten used to? Is it something you've developed as a defence mechanism or to hide? Is it holding you back from achieving your ultimate goal and dreams?

If any of the above is true, then it really isn't you. It's a mask and it's time to discard it.

I mentioned earlier about living in a box. We all have boxes. Some are larger than others, but we all have a limit, a place where our mind says "NO, STOP!" It's called our Comfort Zone. We all have one. The fun is pushing it and making it bigger!

The funny thing about living in a box is that while we can only see the inside, everyone else can only see the outside. Others often see where we are stopping ourselves better than we can. Why is that? It's because they are on the outside looking in. On a box of rice, there are instructions. If you were inside the box, you wouldn't be able to see the instructions and would wonder what to do with these hard little pellets. They certainly don't seem edible inside the box. Those outside the box can easily tell you what to do with the rice, if you're willing to listen. Then you can create a beautiful dish, add some veggies, shrimp and spices and make a yummy dinner. Until you are willing to see things from a different perspective, you will be stuck in the same old viewpoint.

We all have filters. We see the world through our experiences, what we've been told by others and our own thoughts. These create a distortion and often prevent us from seeing things clearly. Our minds only know what they know. It will go over and over the same thing and come up with the same conclusions every time. You've heard the definition of insanity – doing the same thing over and over, expecting different results. Or "If you do what you've always done, you'll get what you've always gotten." If you want things to change, you need to look outside your filters and be willing to see things from the perspective of others.

THE BAD KITTY'S TAIL:

Compared with some of the stories I've told you so far, this may seem trivial. It's a great example of how we look at things one way and can change our view if we're willing to look with new eyes. It can be something apparently small or huge and life changing. I feel even the small things can be life changing, as any change of perspective has ripple effects.

I always hated my ass. I thought it was flat and full of cellulite. When I released 20 pounds a couple of years ago, I hated it even more. A lot of women lose weight off their chest; I lost a lot on my rear. I had a terrible time finding pants to fit because my butt was smaller and they would bag in the back. Eventually I found some styles that fit. They are out there for everyone!

I met someone who loved my behind and told me so repeatedly. "You have a great ass," he'd say as he gave it a smack. At first I just laughed it off. Ya, right, whatever! Eventually I heard it enough from him, and others, that I began to believe it. Now when I look in the mirror I see a great ass.

Something so seemingly insignificant changed my sense of self. It shifted my confidence level about my body. It makes me smile when I'm told, "Did you know that guy watched you as walked past?" Rather than being surprised, I'm flattered and think, "Well, why wouldn't he?"

For my birthday this last year I got a card that said "Just a note to let you know..... You have a great ass." I could honestly say, "Thank you!" rather than being embarrassed and thinking they were just being nice and grabbed the first card they could find.

Seeing yourself through the eyes of others is valuable. It gives such a different perspective and can create a huge shift in how you see yourself.

BAD KITTY SCRATCHING POST:

I've worked with many women who have body issues. They don't want to get naked in front of anyone, not even their husbands. They think they are less valuable because they're not "perfect". They are always comparing themselves to others unfavourably.

Does any of this sound familiar?
The funny thing is, almost everyone has something about their body they're unhappy with.

I have had women stand in front of a group of other women and have asked them to strip down to their underwear. They then point to what they don't like about their bodies. There are usually many spots. I then ask the other women in the group to do the same from their places.

It is a powerful moment when all of these women look back at the woman at the front with love and acceptance and show what body parts they aren't happy with. Even the skinny ones, the fit ones, the seemingly "perfect" ones point at something they don't like.

This is a moment for the woman at the front to see through different eyes. To see all of these women she has been getting to know be willing to be vulnerable in support of her. To see that we all have issues with our bodies. And most of all, to see that we are all beautiful in our diversity.

Go back to chapter 3 and read about Jamie Lee Curtis and her magazine article.

Another powerful way to deal with body issues is with pole dancing. I am always amazed and inspired at how women view themselves differently just from learning a few moves on the pole. They get the opportunity to really feel their Sensuality. It comes alive on the pole no matter what their size, shape or body image.

One woman, Dara Lee, is a great example of this. She says, "Hey, it's me, whose feet don't leave the ground. I just wanted to thank you for doing the pole dancing lessons. I've noticed a difference in myself right from how I walk to how I think of my body. Even my husband has noticed a change! It's amazing how pole dancing has made me feel sexy, even after 3 kids!"

The willingness to see things through new eyes can make all the difference. Are you willing to see things from outside the box and without your filters?

BAD KITTY SCRATCHING POST:

Send the following email out to at least 20 people today. Do a variety of people from different areas of your life; friends, family, co-workers, business associates, classmates. Be open to their answers. Some of them may surprise you! Look for patterns. If you see something over and over that is something you don't see in yourself that surprises you, take a closer look at it.

WARNING: You will not hear back from every-one. DO NOT TAKE THIS PERSONALLY!!! DO NOT MAKE UP STORIES ABOUT WHY THEY DIDN'T RESPOND! You don't know what's going on in their life. You don't know if they even opened the email. You don't know what's going on at the other end, so don't make yourself crazy over it! Concentrate on the ones who did respond and be sure to thank them.

Email to send:

Hi (fill in name)

I am reading a book called "THE BAD KITTY HANDBOOK." I have reached a portion of the book where I have been asked to see myself through the eyes of others. The concept is that sometimes it's easy to get wrapped up in my own views and opin-ions which may not be true to those around me. I may not see myself accurately at all. I would love to know how you see me!

I value your opinion and would greatly appreci-ate it if you would help me see myself in a new light. Please reflect on your experience of me and answer the questions below. If possible, please respond within the next week? Thank you.

What qualities and characteristics do you most admire or respect in me? (Note: These are things about me as a person, my style, personality, values etc.)

1.

2.

3.

What <u>natural abilities or talents</u> do you see in me - tasks or activities where I consistently perform with excellence? (Note: These are things I do extremely well and they seem to come easily to me.)

1.

2.

3.

In your opinion, <u>what am I am most passionate about</u>? What energizes me? (Note: These are specific activities and tasks that I am drawn to and make me come alive.)

1.

2.

3.

If you could use one word or phrase to describe me, what would it be?

Feel free to give any other feedback on your experience of me.

Thank you very much for your support and assistance. Please return this by email to (fill in your email address).

Sincerely,

(Your name)

How does it feel to even contemplate getting feedback from others? Does it create some fear? Good! It can be intimidating to open yourself up to such honest feedback. You may be thinking of all the bad things you're sure they're going to say about you. You may be afraid that they actually DO see you even though you try so hard to hide. You may alternately think that to them, as much as you want to be seen, you really are as invisible as you've always suspected.

These are exactly the reasons you need to do this, or something similar, on a regular basis. These thoughts are all part of your filters. When we check in with what is actually going on, the results can be quite surprising.

Have you ever thought someone didn't like you and then found out through a friend that they actually really liked you and that's why they were so shy around you? Have you ever thought someone was mad at you but they were actually all wrapped up in something that had happened that had nothing to do with you? Have you ever suspected something was up in a relationship but were too afraid to check it out and then got slapped in the face with it later?

When we actually check into things, our filters clear and we can see things for what they really are. Rather than stewing in the thoughts that Jennifer is mad at me, why not ask Jennifer. Simply go up and say, I have this thought that I've done something that has made you angry, is that true? This will either start a dialogue about a perceived sleight on her part or you may find out that she's just really tired and is in her head about how much she wants a nap.

When you decide NOT to check in on things, they can get way out of hand, either in your own mind or in reality.

THE BAD KITTY'S TAIL:

1. I have had a friend, Tamara, since before I was married. That's a long time in my life. Over the years our contact has become less frequent, but there is still a definite connection. When we do see each other it's as if there hasn't been a 6 month gap and we chat and laugh freely.

Over a year ago, Tamara got married. I was invited to the wedding. I was dating someone at the time. I hadn't seen Tamara for awhile and was feeling crappy the weekend of the wedding, plus my boyfriend wasn't able to make it. I called and left Tamara a message apologizing that I wasn't going to make it to the wedding and wishing her the best.

I didn't hear from her so I assumed she was angry with me.

Many months later I was talking to my sister who does Tamara's hair. She mentioned that Tamara had been asking about me. I said, Oh, I thought she was mad at me. Apparently, Tamara thought the same of me. Through my sister, we reconnected. Had it not been for this intermediary, because neither of us checked in on the reality, our friendship of so many years may have been over. And that would have been very sad.

2. A couple of years after my marriage ended, I met a man 10 years my senior. *Rob was everything I wanted at the time. He was creative – did photography as a hobby and for a small alternate income – he was funny, attentive and a bit of a project. He introduced me to *Peak Potentials* training and T. Harv Eker. He is the reason I started on my growth path and am at this point now.

When we took our first course together, we did a lot of sharing, as the course was designed to drill into your psyche around money. We learned a lot about each other that weekend and at the end of it, he confessed that he loved me. I had been holding back the same sentiment for quite some time. It was a relief to finally be able to say it. The problem was that he was getting on a bus to go home, as we didn't live in the same city at the time, and neither of us had cell phones back then. I had to wait 3 hours before we could talk about the "I Love Yous" that had just been exchanged! How frustrating!

Not long after that, I moved back to Edmonton and we moved in together. As is the case, now that we were at a new level of comfort and intimacy with each other, things slowly changed. I have a tendency of keeping to myself until I'm ready to share. I don't spout off about everything. I'm not your "typical" chatty woman. Rob is more talkative and expected me to be the same. Eventually it started to get to him and he felt I was intentionally not sharing with him. I felt I was sharing, just on my own time.

Things started to fall apart. I could see it, but I refused to acknowledge it. I knew he was cheating, but I refused to take the blindfold off and really see it. The night of his birthday when he came home at 3am was a really good sign! I pretended they were just friends. I thought that things would work themselves out.

As we all know from experience, that doesn't happen. I needed to take off my filters and say in plain language, "I think there's something going on with you and *Sheila. Are you sleeping with her?" Yes, he could have lied. Even in the lie, there are clues, if you're open to really seeing. In the end, he didn't lie. When I finally asked him flat out, he confessed. By that time it was too late. Had I said something when I first saw things going sideways, it may have been saved. Or not, but at least it would have kept us both from months of hiding and heart-ache.

I'm sure you can think of a few examples where you have thought something was true that turned out to not be, or knew something was up and chose to ignore it. We all do it. Sometimes it seems easier to ignore things than face them head on. In the end, it doesn't serve either party involved. Why not be brave and get clear?

BAD KITTY SCRATCHING POST:

It's time to clean up an old conversation or assumption. Think about a situation that you have left hanging for some time. Is it a friend you need to confront about disrespectful behaviour? Maybe you think a co-worker hates you; it's time to find out. Are you holding onto something a parent did to you in childhood? Talk to them about it, maybe their remembrance is completely different. Is there someone you're attracted to that you need to tell so you can act normal around them? Is your child doing something out of character that you need to check out?

It can be hard to really look at these things, but do it anyway. Take a deep breath and think about what you're going to say. Phrase it in as non-judgmental a way as you can. Make it about you, not them. Ask them calmly and clearly about it. Keep breathing and be open to the response. You may be surprised by it!

How did that work out for you? I expect that it wasn't as bad as you made it in your head. You probably found that a lot of things you were thinking were inaccurate. You may have discovered that you see more clearly than you thought. Either way, we always need to be checking in to see what's real.

One thing that is real for all of you, my beautiful Kitties, is you. We are all a mix of fears, confidence, joy, sadness, craziness and being grounded. The question is, what do you want to live in? Do you want to conquer your fears and be more confident? Do you want to have more joy and release the sadness? Do you want to live your dreams rather than letting the crazy thoughts in your head run you?

It's time to own the fact that your good and "bad" work together to create you. All your experiences mix together to make you. It's how you mix it, how you choose to react to it, how you talk to yourself that makes you.

You can choose to see things in a new light. You can choose to focus on the positive. You can choose to release your own filters and see what others see about you. You can choose to be all you that you are inside and all that you have dreamed about. You don't have to stay stuck in your box. The only one keeping you there is you.

Live large! Live you! Get past all the craziness of your head and let loose.

The key to being a BAD KITTY is knowing and loving you in all those fearful, confident, joyful, sad, crazy and grounded moments. It will take some time to adjust your patterns and habits. It will take some time to see through new filters. The changes in perspective won't happen all at once. You will need to be aware of your thoughts and whether they are helping or hurting your ultimate goal.

THAT LITTLE VOICE:

Sometimes I wonder why they call it the "little" voice. If yours is like mine, it can be pretty damn loud! For those of you who may be unsure of what I'm referring to, it's that voice in your head that tells you to stop, that you can't, that it won't work. It's the voice that keeps you in your box.

The voice is not designed to be evil; it's there to keep you safe. It wants to keep you from harm and hurt. It's the one that brings up the red flags when you're in a situation similar to one that's hurt you in the past. It's also one that will keep you from the changes you want to make.

When you're going in a direction that you know is right and all of a sudden a big stop sign appears in your head, that's your little voice. When you're doing affirmations or setting goals, it's the one that says "That won't work" or "Why should it be different this time?" When you go in a new direction and you suddenly get a fear hit, that's the voice.

As I said, it's not inherently evil. There are times when it does good work. Alternatively, when it makes you feel fearful or doubtful it's likely working against you. You need to honour the fact that it's just doing its job to keep you safe, while at the same time letting it know that you're changing your patterns and getting out of that box.

A good way to do this is to simply talk to it. Take a breath and say "Thank you for sharing, but I'm up to something else." You may need to say it several times before the little voice lays off. It will come back, but each time it will be less insistent until your pattern has changed. Then suddenly you'll realize that you haven't heard the voice on that subject in quite some time. In that moment, celebrate! You have made a big shift in your life.

I am speaking from experience here! Not only my own, but that of many others I have witnessed on their journey. I like things to happen fast. I work fast. I think fast. I have no patience for slow. I like games where a turn happens in moments, not minutes. As much fun as foreplay is, I like to get to the main event. I always have the result in mind and can be quite impatient with the process.

Coming from someone like that, believe me when I say, the process is worth it! No, it's not always easy. Yes, it can be frustrating. And you can do it, I swear.

You have it in you. You are you and you are beautiful. No matter your weight, your job, your relationship - you are incredible! Own it and start living the motto, BE BEAUTIFUL, BE YOU.

Now let's discover what it is you want to show to the world. What face have you been hiding? It's time to let it shine. Let's go!

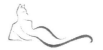

CHAPTER SIX: BAD KITTY LOVE

So far we've looked at the background of Sensuality and why it makes a difference in the way we live our lives. We've seen examples of BAD KITTIES and how they are women of all types. We've seen what works against our Sensuality and why it gets suppressed and repressed. We've taken a look at what you can do to regain what has been lost. So now what?

For many, it's been so long since you've truly loved yourself, you don't even know how. You may even wonder what there is to love, anyway. Life may have beaten you down so badly that you think you're unlovable. You may have been so wrapped up in taking care of others for so long that you can't remember what makes you amazing. There have been so many comparisons to others over the years that you can't see yourself as yourself without anything to measure against.

THE BAD KITTY'S TAIL:

I've made reference earlier to how my sister was called "the pretty one." This is a picture of us. Neither of us generally have dark hair, but we both did at the same time so we took advantage of it by doing some goth pictures. This was taken by photographer Russ Hewitt of Edmonton (used with permission).

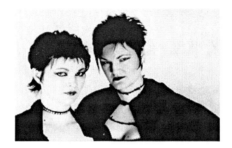

My sister, Shari, is on the left. When others look
at this picture, most say "Wow, you guys look a lot
alike." When she and I look at it, we see the differences. Her face is rounder and softer; lips are fuller,
eyes bigger, turned up nose.

When I look at us now, I still see the differences,
but I also see that we're both pretty hot in our own
ways. That's one great thing about humans, we all
like different things. Those attracted to softness
would pick Shari. Those who like strong features
choose me. Growing up, though, it was a different
story. I grew up thinking I was ugly. Not because
anyone ever said so specifically, but because I always
heard "Oh, she's so cute/pretty/adorable" aimed in
Shari's direction and not mine. Boys noticed her
first. She was the one that modeled when we were
children. She took the dance and baton classes.
She was the girl.

I got so used to the situation that I didn't even
try. I didn't start shaving my legs until late in high
school. I would wear clothes that made me disappear
into the background. I lived all my teen years looking down as I walked the halls watching everyone
else with their boyfriends as I remained dateless.

I used to get quite cynical when watching family
sit-coms. There always seemed to be an episode

wherein the eldest received a speech about how they should be easier on their younger sibling, because as the oldest they got to do everything first. Not in our family. All the big milestones happened to Shari first – boyfriend, period, driver's license, engaged. I was always behind.

It took many years and a lot of work to get over those feelings. Now I get many compliments on my looks – including comments that I'm better looking than my sister. I don't always believe that one, but I can certainly own that I'm just as hot as she is and that I'm smokin'!

We've already talked about filters and how the opinions of others often skew our view of ourselves. The need to look outside what we've already decided is true to find out how things may have changed is critical.

ANOTHER BAD KITTY'S TAIL:

*Arlene was emotionally abused by her husband. After 8 years of hearing that she was ugly, useless and stupid, she believed him. Her usual bright and social personality changed. She became withdrawn and fearful. She watched her every move, hoping not to create an issue.

Eventually, her friends helped her see that for her own sanity, she needed to leave. She started to secretly put away money and make plans. Even in this step she started to become more confident. She knew she wasn't stuck.

Finally, the opportunity came. Her husband was going to be away for a long weekend, camping and quadding. Friends helped her pack and move.

When he came home, she was gone. As soon as she walked out the door, she changed. Her sense of self re-emerged. It was as if a huge weight was lifted and she could breathe again.

After the divorce, there was still some work she wanted to do. She went from working in retail and food services to rediscovering her passion for fashion and became a designer. She took the time to know herself again, before seeking another relationship, and has now been remarried very happily to a man who treats her like gold - whom she respects and loves whole-heartedly.

It takes time for our sense of self and our love of self to be broken, so it also takes time to rebuild. The key is to know that you're worth it and you deserve it. No matter what you've been told by others in the past, either out of good intentions or bad, you are amazing!

THE BAD KITTY'S TAIL:

Being conditioned for so long to think poorly of myself, there are many examples of feedback from others that it took a long time to accept.

The first came from my second boyfriend. I only had one date when I was in high school; the only reason I agreed to go out with him was because his brother was going to be there and I had a crush on him. I didn't have my first "real" boyfriend until I was 19. At that point I was feeling pretty ugly and unlovable because not only had my little sister had several boyfriends by then, she was also engaged! Needless to say, my first choice was not a good one. He was cute – big brown puppy dog eyes – and he liked me. That's all I needed at that time! It was a disaster of a relationship and certainly didn't add to my sense of self love.

The next one was better in some ways. He was charming and popular, smart and full of ideas. During one of our first conversations he told me that men were intimidated by me. This seemed impossible to me. "How?" "You're tall, smart and beautiful and that intimidates most men."

The fact that he called me beautiful was enough to give me pause in how I viewed myself. Add in the rest, which I did already know, and turning me into a triple threat against male confidence was beyond my realm of thought.

It wasn't until I heard similar comments from lovers and friends over the years that I started to see it may actually be true. And now I'm a quad-ruple threat, as I'm confident as well. Thankfully I am also surrounded by people of a different calibre than I was then and men are attracted rather than intimidated. Although there is still some intimida-tion, I'm told. Silly boys. They're so cute!

When I started to do self development work many people, women especially, started to call me an inspiration. Every time I heard that one, for quite some time, I had a hard time taking it in. My brain would go into overload. Me, what, how? I had been invisible for so long I couldn't conceive that some-one would actually look to me as a model.

I now own that responsibility and take it quite seriously. My growth and change and the person I am now is an inspiration – to me and to others. That's one reason I'm writing this book. I realize that who I am now can help others be who they have always wanted to be. It's a big job and I'm proud to do it!

The most recent one I've been receiving is that I'm very authentic. A friend told me just the other day, "You're the most authentic person I've ever known." That's true to her, and the others that have said similar things. It's not that I'm so much better than others. I don't look on it as a point of pride. They see what they see through their filters and that it's true for them so there must be some truth behind it.

What's changed for me is how I receive such feedback. I can now honestly and humbly say "Thank you" rather than going into my head and trying to figure out what it means. Or going into my denial mode and thinking they're just saying that or that they're flawed somehow for thinking such a thing.

How many times have you received a compliment and you brush it off? "This old thing?" "Oh, well, I just ... (fill in your excuse here)." A compliment is a gift. It deserves to be received as such. When you start to accept compliments from others, you will see a difference in the way you feel about what is said.

You may actually start to believe them! You will give a gift back to the giver by being a gracious receiver. You will be more likely to compliment others sincerely. You will want to give back.

BAD KITTY SCRATCHING POST:

Notice how many compliments you get in a day. "I love your hair like that." "That top really suits you." "You did a great job with that customer." "You're a great friend." "You have such a talent with computers." "I could never do that, you make it look so easy." "You're beautiful." "I couldn't have done it without you." "I love that necklace." "That was a great meal."

They come from everywhere and from all kinds of people. It could be the cashier at the grocery store, your family, friends or a stranger at the mall.

Be aware of these comments or compliments. Notice how you want to minimize them by making excuses or pretending you didn't hear. When you notice yourself doing that, take a moment, look the person in the eye and simply say, "Thank you." Notice the desire to say more, to explain or justify. Leave the thank you as it is. Nothing else is necessary. Anything further deflates the compliment and removes the power of the gift from the giver.

You may even notice yourself getting so used to hearing compliments that you almost forget to be gracious. Many years ago I started putting unnatural colors in my hair – pink, purple, blue. Shari is my hairdresser and is especially talented; I would get compliments almost daily from friends and strangers. It got to the point where I would hear "I love your hair" and wouldn't even look up to make sure they were talking to me, I'd just automatically say "Thank you." It got to the point that my boyfriend started saying "thank you" as a joke.

Be sure to remain sincere in your thanks! Now I always make sure I make eye contact and smile. I want to give back to the giver with a true thank you and not a knee jerk reaction.

Doing these seemingly little things will help you fall back in love with yourself. It's easy to look outside of ourselves for validation. It's easy to look around for the acceptance of others in order to be more accepting of ourselves. It does help, but the true love must come from inside. The attention of others will wax and wane. For every one that comes to build you up, someone or something else will tear you down – most often by omission rather than deliberately.

How many times have you dressed up and thought you looked amazing and no one said anything? How many times have you been attracted to someone and had them not return the sentiment? How many times have you looked to a friend for a much needed boost in esteem and they were too wrapped up in what was going on in their own lives to notice? How many times have you looked at your bank account, wondered where the money went and got down on yourself? How many times have you applied for a job or called a customer where you thought you were a shoo-in and were instead rejected?

Unless you are internally secure in yourself, these things can ruin your day, your week and/or your life if you let them. There will always be outside forces you can't control. If you let the outside rule you, you won't get very far.

THE BAD KITTY'S TAIL:

Having had so little attention from men when I was younger, and wanting it so badly, I have been ruled by the need for validation by men for a long time.

Even recently, I saw that tendency raise its ugly head. It's fun to be human and to remember that no matter what, we are not perfect. Yes, things are multitudes better than they were, but I still find when I'm feeling especially out of my element, the old patterns can seep back in.

I was at an event in Lake Tahoe and there were hundreds of people there. In the past I would have been completely intimidated by that fact and stuck close to the ones I knew. I am now more willing to venture out, to start conversations with strangers and the "I can't mingle" tape I used to play is all but erased.

Still, it was a new situation. A lot of new information was flying around. New expectations were levied. I watched others do their thing and fell into the trap of comparison. I was spiritually open and became overwhelmed by the support and information on many occasions. I have been in many groups that were supportive and loving, but never of this magnitude. It nearly blew my circuits.

My pattern is to find solace in the company of men. Since I have discovered my comfort and power as a woman, that's usually not very difficult. As we discussed before, I am a quadruple threat (tall, beautiful, smart and confident). I say this not out of pride. It's a fact I've come to accept as true from the observations and feedback of others. It's part of who I am. I don't use it against men or hold it over anyone's head. I simply recognize that I can be intimidating and am sure to watch for signs of it. I'm also open and caring which people recognize and are drawn to despite the intimidation factor some feel.

That said, I'm used to both being avoided by men and attracting them. At this event, I made several male friends, all of whom I thought were great fun, very sweet and incredible people – and some were single. I also watched many of my single friends hook up while I didn't. There occurred over the weekend a moment or three where I disengaged because I was getting that old feeling of not being wanted.

I hate having that one come back! And yet, I am in control. I took the time to recognize that I was slipping back into old habits. I took a moment to speak to my little voice and thank it for sharing. I took the time to notice all the valuable relationships I had made with men and women. I was thankful for those people and the time they took to get to know me and give of themselves.

THE KEY:

We've discussed the inner little voice. We've discussed filters. It's valuable to be aware of all of these things and dealing with them contributes to building your personal confidence and power.

Loving yourself – even in moments of weakness - is the key to your Sensuality and to your BAD KITTY-ness.

There are a number of things to do when you notice the old patterns kicking in.
- Recognize it. Call it what it is, make no excuses.
- Be aware of how you would normally handle it and choose to do it another way.
- Notice what you can be thankful for in the situation.
- Celebrate that you are changing a pattern and that you are growing.

We often forget the last step. Celebration is integral! A pat on the back, a moment to breathe and smile. A little "yippee", a high five, a laugh. Get an "Easy" button and push it. Take the time to let your successes sink in.

Success is a key to loving yourself. It's important to find ways to impress yourself. Doing something as seemingly insignificant as being on time is a moment for celebration.

- Take those negative thoughts about yourself and do something different that proves it wrong.
- Notice when you do something well and acknowledge it.
- Do something that you're afraid of.
- Do something that you think you're not good at.
- Do something that's out of your comfort zone.
- Be in the moment rather than multi-tasking.
- Take a moment to make someone else's day.
- Finish something that's been hanging over your head for a long time.
- Spend a moment with your child rather than saying "later" for the third time.
- Accomplish something on your dream list.
- Let a friend pick something she feels will push you.

The list is endless! There are myriads of ways you can impress yourself every day.

Nothing adds to your BAD KITTY love more than doing things that surprise you. Make sure to acknowledge and celebrate those moments. You are incredible and you just proved it, so take the time to really feel. Taking that time ingrains it in you.

BAD KITTY SCRATCHING POST:

Every day, ask yourself this simple question - "What can I do in this situation that will cause me to be impressed with myself?" Use it over and over throughout the day. It can be while you're waiting in traffic. It can be with your children. It can be during a disagreement with your husband. It can be during a conversation with a friend. It can be in conjunction with the time you get up or go to bed. It can be about taking a moment for you. The possibilities are endless.

Get yourself a pretty notebook and take it out every night. Keep an "Impress Yourself" journal. Go through your day and recall the moments when you did something – small or large – that caused you to smile, feel a lift in your spirit and, ultimately, to feel good about yourself. Make an effort to recognize at least 3 things every day.

Be aware, it's easy to pretend that something we did was no big deal or to minimize it. Sometimes our brain has a hard time dealing with how fabulous we are because it's so conditioned to keep you small.

ANOTHER BAD KITTY'S TAIL:

I took part in an event many years ago that had a fire walk. For those of you who have never done a fire walk, it is an incredible experience. To walk across coals in your bare feet is quite intimidating – and exciting, once you get to the other side. A word of warning – if you decide to try a fire walk - be sure to do so with qualified pit builders as the mix of wood, depth of coals and other factors are extremely important to your safety.

At this event we all stood around the track. I could feel the heat blasting my face from 10 feet away. The pit tenders were wearing bandanas and welders gloves up their elbows. They were covered with soot. The tension in the air was palpable. The procedure was to choose someone to meet you on the other side of the pit to celebrate your crossing with you. You set an intention out loud before walking and strolled - no running, tiptoeing or meandering, walk at a normal pace – across the coals.

A friend of mine who was there, *Mel, reported to me the next day. Like me, Mel had felt a great sense of accomplishment after walking the coals. It was a self esteem boost. Then her head started to do a number on her. "Well, it's not really that hot. Everyone else is doing it so it can't be so difficult. There's some sort of trick."

After the walk was over, Mel returned to her room and washed her feet. In that moment she realized it was no trick. She had been wearing a band aid on the sole of her foot. It was now fused into her skin. Yes, it really was that hot! Her head wanted to keep the experience small, to make it safe to discount the power of it so she wouldn't have to live up to the power the experience gave her.

BAD KITTY SCRATCHING POST:

Take your notebook. Find your quiet space. Think of a time when you accomplished something that you were especially impressed with. Something that made you so excited to share, something that made you feel your most powerful and confident. Record this event and how it made you feel in that moment.

What happened afterwards? Did someone else say something that caused you to minimize the event? Did you somehow talk yourself down to make it less in your own mind? How does it feel to compare the initial empowerment to the way you then downplayed it?

Think again about the initial feeling you had. Sit with it. Let it flow over you. THAT is the reality of the situation. THAT is the one that you want to hold in your mind and heart. When the thoughts that minimize it come up, thank your little voice and move on.

Record how your life would be different if you lived in that feeling of power and accomplishment at all times. How would you handle your relationships differently? Maybe there are some people you would remove or limit contact with in your life. Would there be a difference in the direction you take in your life? Would your income be different? How would you carry yourself? How would you express yourself? Would you be bolder, braver, more willing to take a risk? Would you be more peaceful, joyful and engaged in life?

TRUE SELF:

Being truly in love with you is a tricky prospect. I'm sure a number of you have already had the thought, perhaps more than once, that this is pride. It's wrong to feel too highly of yourself.

Please allow me a moment to speak my mind without reservation – BULLSHIT!

Knowing your own strengths and beauty and being aware that you are incredible is not pride in the way that many think of it. Many see pride by this definition: "A high or inordinate opinion of one's own dignity, importance, merit, or superiority, whether as cherished in the mind or as displayed in bearing, conduct, etc" (dictionary.com).

This is an out of proportion way of seeing yourself that leads to seeing others as less than yourself. It's a way of feeling superior by seeing others as inferior. This is unhealthy. It's also untrue. People that have this type of pride don't have true love of self. It's like a bully who asserts their physicality to make themselves feel better. This type of pride is a way of asserting a perceived superiority by way of ignoring the things that make them feel less confident or powerful.

True pride comes from a grounded, realistic sense of self; "A becoming or dignified sense of what is due to oneself or one's position or character; self-respect; self-esteem" (dictionary.com).

Pride that comes from a healthy sense of esteem; where you know your strengths and are unafraid to face your fears and challenges creates a completely different dynamic. It lets people in and recognizes that we all have our struggles. It is the true and complete expression of self. It draws people to you instead of pushing them away. It is confidence that doesn't require making others feel small in order to be felt. It's recognizing and loving your essence, your true self, your Sensuality.

Many of us have grown up with the instruction to be modest. Don't stand out. Don't brag. Don't draw attention to yourself.

I'm here to say STOP IT!!! You have every right to show your light, to stand out in a crowd, to know your skills, talents and what makes you unique and to share it with the world.

Many of you have probably heard Marianne Williamson's quote, but let me share it with you again:

"Our deepest fear is not that we are inadequate. Our deepest fear is that we are powerful beyond measure. It is our light, not our darkness that most frightens us. We ask ourselves, Who (sic) am I to be brilliant, gorgeous, talented, fabulous? Actually, who are you *not* to be? You are a child of God. Your playing small does not serve the world. There is nothing enlightened about shrinking so that other people won't feel insecure around you. We are all meant to shine, as children do. We were born to make manifest the glory of God that is within us. It's not just in some of us; it's in everyone. And as we let our own light shine, we unconsciously give other people permission to do the same. As we are liberated from our own fear, our presence automatically liberates others."

This is what being a BAD KITTY is all about. Truly loving yourself and letting it shine to the world. A BAD KITTY embraces every part of herself. She loves her light, she's aware of her dark. She knows she has a little naughtiness and lets it out when it serves her.

Ladies, admit it:
- You want to let loose.
- You want to live large.
- You want to be FREE.

Instead of being worried about approval, about doing it "right" and being "good" it's time to be BAD and make a difference!

Loving yourself gives you permission to free yourself. It gives you the power to live your dreams and goals. It gives you the joy that has come in fits and spurts in your life. It gives you the deep down knowledge that no matter what anyone else says or does to you, you are INCREDIBLE.

I don't even know you and I love you. I know that under your insecurities, the extra weight you hate, the fear that rules you – underneath it all you are beautiful and powerful beyond even your wildest dreams.

I KNOW THIS WITHOUT QUESTION OR RESERVATION!

What's been stopping you from recognizing it in yourself?

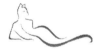

CHAPTER SEVEN:GOING OUT WITH THE BAD KITTY

We've discussed that there is a difference between Sensuality and Sexuality. In no section of this book is this more true than this one; how do you use your Authentic Sensuality in your day to day life?

Since Sensuality is your Senses and the culmination of who we all are as individuals, the easy answer is EVERYWHERE in EVERY SITUATION!

TOUCH, TOUCH, FEEL:

Recently a tissue commercial came out with a woman going through her life. The word "touch" is used each time she reaches out for something – the elevator button, the clock, and her clothes – until she reaches for the tissue box. In that moment she stops, smiles and the word changes to "FEEL". She even steals the box.

That is Sensuality. In every moment of your life you are taking a moment to FEEL. We usually live in the touch, touch, touch mode. We live on the surface, not really taking the time to really interact or even notice the people and things around us.

I read a restaurant review recently where the reviewer said that there is a difference between "eating out" and "going out for dinner." Eating out is getting food and not really caring about the experience. Going out for dinner is when you really enjoy the experience in all aspects from the food to the environment. It's easy to "eat out" even when you're in a nice place if you're not really present. It's easy to "go out for dinner" at home as long as you are enjoying the company, the food and the environment.

- How many times have you chosen to eat something fast in the car rather than sitting down and enjoying a meal?

- How many times have you filled your day so full that you were rushing from one thing to another, barely leaving time to breathe? Actually, let me ask, when is the last time you DIDN'T do that?

- How many times have you been having a conversation with a friend and you realize 10 minutes in that you weren't even listening?

- How many times have you yelled at your child or spouse or been short with a stranger simply because you were feeling stress and weren't dealing with it?

THE BAD KITTY'S TAIL:

I'm hypoglycaemic. For those of you unfamiliar with the term, it means I'm prone to low blood sugar. If I don't eat regularly it causes me to get shaky, become unfocused and grumpy. It's not the same as diabetes. Diabetics create little or no insulin that regulates blood sugar and need to use injections to regulate it. I only need food.

An unfortunate side effect of this is that some-times I wait too long to eat. Sometimes it's out of my control. For example, once I was at a meeting that was supposed to end at noon. They had supplied snacks, but of course they were high sugar snacks which don't last or satisfy the body. The meeting ended after 1. I had no vehicle and was at the mercy of others as to when we got to a restaurant. I was fighting to control what I knew was going on in my body, but it can only be fought for so long. When we finally got seated at Olive Garden where, of course, there was a wait, I was on the verge of snapping. The server came to the table and I said "I'm hypo-glycaemic and I'm starting to get the shakes. I need breadsticks – NOW." I guess I was a little intense as everyone at the 15 person table was paying atten-tion. The other problem is, when I do finally get the food, I eat too fast and don't enjoy it.

Having this condition can make it so that I don't really enjoy my meals. I often am eating simply to stop the inevitability of my body reacting to low blood sugar.

When I was in New Orleans I had another mem-orable reaction. I was in a group looking for a res-taurant along Bourbon Street. I was already get-ting punchy as, when you're in a group of women, things don't always run smoothly. We had to wait for several of our party to "get ready" and left the hotel half an hour later than planned. As we walked along I was getting more and more irritated and my hand was starting to shiver. Finally at the fourth restaurant where everyone was looking at the menu and hemming and hawing I said firmly – and prob-ably a little loudly - "Just pick something already!" We went in.

Apart from that incident, New Orleans was a time when I enjoyed every moment - especially the food. I'm not a big seafood or fish fan. In NOLA, everything tastes wonderful! I enjoyed crawfish my first night. I had BBQ shrimp, turtle soup, grilled gator, and redfish – everyday I had something I might hesitate to order anywhere else. Every meal – except the grits I had for breakfast one morning – was truly amazing. I took the time to savour each bite. That, as much as the quality of the food, contributed to my favourable memory of it.

When I travel, I enjoy everything more. I take time to really see, to really notice all the details around me. I could never do a cruise or tour. I like to take my time. When in San Diego I took a full day at locations that they give you a couple hours to see on a tour.

I am fully Sensual on vacation. I am fully in the moment with very little agenda.

It's easier to be fully present on vacation because we don't have to worry about the day to day things. It takes a little more concentration to do it day to day, but it is possible.

Life is full of opportunities to experience. We've become so used to being in our own little worlds with our cell phones and iPods, computers and TV's, take out or delivery and drive thru that it's easy to be isolated. We have become very separate from life. Nature is something "out there." Many have become uncomfortable with something as simple as eye contact. We stand apart from each other rather than connecting. Food has become generic. Life doesn't have the spark and joy it can have most days due to our holding back and sitting apart.

BAD KITTY SCRATCHING POST:

There are so many ways you can live your life with more Sensuality. Here are 12 suggestions. Take a suggestion each week and try it on. See how differently you view the world when you take the time to FEEL.

- Take a walk without your phone or iPod, preferably in nature.
- Eat at the table without the TV.
- Practice the art of listening.
- Make dinner – from scratch.
- Dress in clothes that make you feel wonderful.
- Make eye contact with people when you're talking to them – and smile.
- Do something creative – draw, paint, write, scrapbook.
- Read for pleasure.
- Go out with friends and leave the cell phone behind.
- Go about your whole day without anything in your ear – iPod, Bluetooth, etc.
- Spend time playing with children.
- Go to a coffee shop without your phone, iPod or book and people watch.

Remember to Journal your experiences. Some will cause a level of discomfort as it'll be something you're not used to. Work through that discomfort and see what's on the other side. You may actually want to create a new habit!

For more suggestions, go to www.thebadkitty/ products.html and purchase my two eBooks. One is 30 sensual tips – one a day for a month. The other is 12 tips requiring more time or preparation – one a month for a year. See the back of the book for a special offer on these eBooks!

MISSING OUT:

Living in your Authentic Sensuality is about truly being in the world and experiencing it. It's also about your Self Expression and being willing to show up as yourself in all situations. It can be easy to hold back, to feel things out, and to make sure you feel "safe" before truly showing yourself. My question to you is how many things have you missed out on because of that habit? How many times has fear stopped you? How many times have you just not been present and didn't see an opportunity for friendship, love or beauty?

These questions are hard to answer because how do you know what you missed. If you missed it, it's gone. So let's take another angle – how much richer would your life be if you showed up in every moment? How much more fun would it be if you dove right in rather than waiting? How many fabulous experiences would you have if you didn't let fear stop you?

ANOTHER BAD KITTY'S TAIL:

I met a woman at an event in Lake Tahoe. Stephanie is a bright, fun, outgoing woman. However, she had a habit of thinking before acting. She came to my condo for a pole dancing lesson. Yes, I took my pole. It was fun showing up with a gun case, which carries the pole, at security! When it came time to spin, Stephanie had a hard time getting up the nerve. It took several turns around the pole before she finally jumped in. Here are her thoughts.

"I had a great experience working with Christie. I went in figuring, at the very least, that I would have some fun and try something new that I had always somewhat guiltily and secretly been interested in trying. Despite my inner voice convincing me otherwise, I cautiously attempted a couple of moves- most notably the fireman's swing which requires lifting both feet off the ground and swinging around the pole. I was petrified to even try, circling the pole on foot a bazillion times before even coming close. While just thinking about trying it was very cool at the time, my real breakthrough came the next morning.

As I was getting dressed, I noticed that I had been singing just the title line of the song "Dear Prudence" over and over again in my head. What was my mind trying to tell me!? I started to laugh and cry simultaneously (my typical reaction to figuring something out about myself).

I realized that I have been too cautious with my body, and I need to take care of it, so that it can do for me what I need and we can have a trusting relationship. Holy smokes, this from a kid who used to count '1-2-3-4, 1-2-3 go' just so that I would have more time to psych myself into doing something. This from the woman who has mistreated and mistrusted her body for over 20 years.

Then the next line of the song came into mind "... won't you come out to play?" and I decided that that was where I want to live my life. Thanks to the fireman's swing and Christie's wonderful encouragement, I had a really fundamental shift in my thinking about and relationship to my body. I gained a lot of confidence, and am getting reacquainted with my body more and more each day. Oh, and by the way, the next time I tried the swing, I got off the ground smiling!"

Stephanie learned a fundamental lesson – love yourself and take a risk. You never know what might happen as a result!

THE BAD KITTY'S TAIL:

I used to live a life of fear. I was afraid to try things, to look foolish, to be misunderstood. As I've mentioned before, I was invisible. Yet, it seemed that when I wasn't invisible I was doing something I was embarrassed by like saying something out of turn or inappropriate.

Once I was in a van with my church youth group. There was one guy there I had a crush on. Being inexperienced and self conscious, I wasn't very good at expressing such things. A conversation began about Saskatchewan, where I'm from. The others were jabbering about how flat it is and so on. The guy I liked made a comment and I threw a pillow at him. It ended up hitting him very hard and awkwardly in the face. The fun abruptly ended and I was given many a dirty look. After a few moments of standing out, I shrank back in.

It wasn't until I became clear on who I was and wasn't continually concerned about whether or not I was the right person for each situation that these awkward situations stopped happening. I can still make faux pas, the difference is how I handle them.

Before I would shrink and be plagued by the thoughts of my perceived stupidity. Now I apologize, learn and move on. I would be embarrassed by attention, now I take it in stride. I was trying to please everyone, now I please myself by knowing who I am in every situation.

I was out for my birthday this year with girl-friends. We went to a chocolate buffet. Yes, really, a chocolate buffet. Now you know what to do for your birthday with your friends! The location of the buffet is a hotel in downtown Edmonton. It is in their tavern which is in the middle of the lobby and has no walls, only railings. We were sitting right next to the rails on the check in desk side of the lobby.

As can often happen when you get 8 women together, it got a little rambunctious. We talked about my upcoming role in a production of "The Vagina Monologues." One part of the show is the demonstration of different types of moans that women do while in pleasure. I was asked which moan I had so I decided to perform it.

It is called the "Mutant Bisexual Moan". I wish I could send you a recording. Let's suffice to say, it's loud and there's no way I could do it softly. A few minutes after the laughter and shock of my moan drifted away, a hotel employee came over to ask that we keep it down because the girl at the front desk couldn't concentrate.

We all laughed and agreed to be more aware of our noise level. We were more respectful of our environment. And we didn't feel bad about having fun.

WORDS AND YOUR EXPRESSION:

This is where things can get touchy. There are many people out there that say, "this is me, if you don't like it, too bad." That is true to an extent. Not everyone is going to like you, so why worry about it. However, that's no excuse for acting like an ass.

A person who is living Authentic Self Expression and Sensuality is respectful of others. For example, I no longer have a hang up about swearing. I believe that words are words. They only have the meaning we put on them. If we react strongly to a word, it has power. If we just consider it a collection of letters, we have the power.

I saw an excellent cartoon once regarding the big F word (used with permission of Stephen Notley).

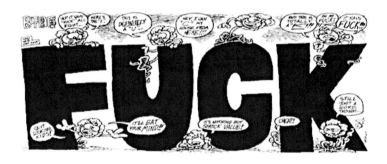

I'm sure a lot of people freaked out when they saw the above, however, check out the last balloon bubble – "still just a word though." It's a collection of letters that we've arbitrarily decided is nasty.

Still, I won't use certain words in front of my mother or children. It would upset my mom and is inappropriate around children. It's not something that's that important to my core expression so I can leave it aside in certain situations. I, personally, don't have any problem with "bad" words; however some do so I respect that. If, however, no other word expressed what needed to be said, I may use it with only a small apology.

What it boils down to is knowing that you are so solid in who you are that you can still respect others while being true to yourself. Only you know if you are acting authentically in any given situation. You can feel it. There is a definite shift in your comfort and presence level.

THE BAD KITTY'S TAIL:

There are still times, even being the teacher and having been so aware over the years, that I find myself slipping. No matter how "in tune" one may get, we are still human.

As I've gotten clearer on who I am, I've gotten more confident. I used to be so terribly insecure because I never knew how to act from one situation to the next that I stayed inside myself unless I was feeling especially bold. I am an introvert; however I am not as shy now that I know my true nature. When you become clear on your Authentic Self you may discover that your own shyness (however you experience it) dissipates. Or it may not. Everyone is different and their true expression will be different. One thing is certain, you will be more confident when you know yourself.

There are so many situations I could share with you about how I've gone in feeling unsettled and unsure and went into my old stand by "shy" place. Recently I went to a party. I got there late and only knew 2 people there well. In the past, I would have been completely intimidated in that scenario. I did go to an apprehensive place beforehand, so much so that I almost didn't go. All the "what if's" came up in my head.

What if I don't know anyone? What if I make a fool of myself? What if I don't like anyone there? What if no one likes me! What if I have nothing to say? What if they find me boring or stupid or just ignore me all together?

And, as is usually the case, all the what if's were just in my head. I was a little quiet for the first 5 minutes or so. Then I made a decision and got involved. I got out of my head and enjoyed myself. Staying in your head is the killer! I was myself, I didn't hold back and I got to know people. That's so much more fun than sitting in the corner worrying about what I should do, when I should do it and if it's the right thing to do in the first place!

So how do you know if you're being Authentic in the moment and sharing your Sensuality with the world? Ask yourself:
- Am I in my head?
- Am I worried about how I will be perceived?
- Am I holding back?
- Am I thinking in the past or the future rather than the present?
- Am I stumbling over my words?
- Am I breathing shallowly?
- Am I ignoring what I sense/perceive about what is going on?
- Am I multi tasking?

It's so easy to pull back and live in the "safe" place. That, unfortunately, is also the land of regrets. I'd rather not live my life wishing, I'd rather be doing. What about you?

BAD KITTY SCRATCHING POST:

Make a list of at least 50 things you want for yourself that are strictly selfish. These have nothing to do with your children, significant other, friends or family. They are for YOU. Your brain may be saying, "FIFTY! What is she nuts?"

Yes, I mean it. FIFTY. I really want you to stretch your mind. They can be very simple like buying sexy underwear to more complex like creating your own business.

Do this exercise quickly. Take only 10 minutes. This will stop you from thinking and analyzing. Let the ideas flow without editing. Don't worry if you think they're doable or practical. Just write them down. Let them build. If some are similar, put it down anyway. Just keep going. If you get more than 50, more power to ya!

Once you have your list, pick two you can do right away and one you want to work on long term. Make a plan to accomplish them. Celebrate your successes along the way. Notice how great it makes you feel to work on something just for you.

The key to truly living your Authenticity and being Sensual is to know what you want; to be willing to speak your mind. To live in a way that allows you to overcome your fear.

As we've discussed, Sensuality is everything about you – how you are in the world. If you are holding back, ignoring your intuition, disregarding your feelings, you cannot be Sensual because you are not Authentic.

AXIOMS:

One key to living authentically is to stop blaming; being the victim or ignoring what is really going on. Our society is so geared to the blame game. It's taken away our ownership as well as our power over our lives.

How many times have you heard, or said:
- It's my mom's fault.
- If my husband had treated me better, I wouldn't be like this.
- Everyone treats me badly.
- You're making me so angry.
- My life stinks because I can't get a good job.
- Things just happen, I can't help it.
- I can't have a good relationship because my whole family is messed up.
- I'm late because of the traffic.

And many more excuses for why we do things, are the way we are or feel the way we feel.

I have good news for you – you are in complete control of it all! Our circumstances only control us as much as we allow them. Have you ever heard of a little something called choice? Yes, we do have it in every situation.

But I have no control over traffic! Yes, you're right. You do have a choice in how you react to it. You have a choice in checking the traffic report before you leave and knowing to leave extra time during rush hour.

But I have no control over how my parents raised me! Yes, you're right. You do have a choice in how you live your life, whether you use your experiences to grow or be stuck, whether you see things in a positive or negative light, whether you decide to move on and leave the pain behind.

But I have no control over what others do to me!
Yes, you're right. You do have a choice in whether
you allow them to treat you poorly. You have a
choice in your reactions. You decide if you stay in
a state of anger, irritation and victimhood or if you
move away from it.

There is ALWAYS a choice!
Hundreds of years ago a philosopher created
three axioms for living a life of choice.

- A THING IS WHAT IT IS
    We label things. We call the thing we sit
    on a chair. What is it really? Two pieces of
    wood nailed together at a 90ish degree angle
    with four sticks nailed to the bottom corners
    of one of the pieces. Its wood, varnish or paint,
    nails and glue. These things are what it truly
    is at the most basic level.
    We label emotions. Sometimes we feel
    queasy in the stomach, tingly in the skin, a
    little light headed and, depending on the situ-
    ation, we label it nervous or excited. Actually,
    the feeling is exactly the same; it's just what
    we decide to call it.
    The first axiom is about simply seeing
    things as they are at the most basic. No labels,
    no layering of expectation or distortion from
    those filters we talked about before. See it for
    what it really is.

- OWN IT AND BE RESPONSIBLE FOR IT AS
    IT IS
    For the chair, it is solid. If you try to punch
    it, you will hurt your hand. If you turn it on its
    side and step on one of the legs, it will prob-
    ably break. Trying to sit on the pokey side will
    hurt or at least not be terribly comfortable. If

you throw it at the wall, it may break and the wall will certainly be worse for wear.

When you are in a situation that starts to push some buttons emotionally, realize you are allowing yourself to feel as you feel. Someone else isn't "making" you angry, you are simply angry. Own that emotion. It's yours. The situation may bring up some things that you haven't dealt with or remind you of another time when similar emotions occurred. And they are YOUR emotions. Own it and be responsible for it. No one can "make" you feel anything. It's your very own special feeling.

- CREATE WHAT YOU WANT
We may call that collection of planks and sticks a chair, but it can be so much more! It can be a space ship, throw a blanket over it and make a fort, a step stool, a zoo for your stuffed animals, part of a maze. You are only limited by your imagination. Ask any child what possibilities there are to create from a chair and you'll be astounded by the ideas. How many kids will put a toy aside and play with the box it came in? That is creating what you want. The box has way more possibilities!

When it comes to emotions, it can be a little trickier until you get the hang of it. To clarify, it's not about being enlightened and somehow above feeling. That's skipping to the end of the process and it will eventually come back and bite your ass. Rather, it's about acknowledging the feeling – step 2 – rather than glossing over it or pretending it doesn't exist or that you're somehow above or better than the emotions, especially the ones we deem "negative" like anger.

In truth, no emotion is negative; it's what you do with it that can have poor consequences. So take how you're feeling, own it and then decide what you are going to do with it. Are you going to channel it in a way that serves or hurts you? Are you going to decide to sit and stew in it or express it and be done with it? It's up to you.

THE BAD KITTY'S TAIL:

A year ago, my boyfriend of a year and a half dumped me without warning. It was a "nice" break up, as break ups go. He said that he felt guilty about leading me on, in a sense, because he didn't feel he could ever feel for me what I felt for him. He wasn't sure he could ever love anyone, for that matter. "I like you, we have fun together, but...." kind of break up.

So, A THING IS WHAT IT IS I could have easily started to make up stories or try to figure out his real motives or any number of reactions to the sudden news. Instead, I chose to put the axioms into action and take it at face value – he didn't want to be together, the reason didn't matter, and I was hurt by that. I let it be what it was.

OWN IT AND BE RESPONSIBLE FOR IT. I took my time to process and understand how I felt. It wasn't until weeks later that I realized I was angry with him. I didn't have a strong initial reaction so I thought that there was no anger. But one day I blew up about something trivial with a stranger and took a closer look. Ahhh, there it was, the anger unexpressed and hiding under all kinds of "enlightenment" about only being hurt. Once I recognized it, I could deal with it and CREATE WHAT I WANTED.

Once I knew I was angry and was responsible for that anger, I was able to deal with it. Until then it was a festering sore just waiting to come out when I – and those around me – least expected it. I did some journaling, talked to some friends and soon it had gone away and changed into first a sadness at the end of a relationship to a fond memory of time spent with a good man who showed me that there were men out there like what I wanted and that I didn't have to settle for anything less.

SENSUAL SEXUALITY

Some of you may be asking, "This is all well and good, but you said the word sexuality at the beginning of the chapter, so what about the Sexuality part of Sensuality?" Good question. It is part of it, so let's talk about it.

Because Sensuality and Sexuality are so closely related, one of the first parts we women shut down when we go into the overwhelm, martyr state is our Sexuality. It leads to a cascade reaction of shutting everything else down as well. When you're not fully present and feeling in one area, it affects all.

This is a big subject and could be a book in itself. Let's do our best to keep it simple. Sex is a super-charged subject in our society. Mention homosexuality, pre-marital sex, extra-marital sex, fetishes, prostitution or anything else to do with the larger subject of sex, and you're bound to get a lively reaction. People will be immediately engaged and wanting to express opinions, others will shut down and want to change the subject. No matter what, there will be a reaction.

In reality, it's like the word fuck – it's not inherently a good or bad thing, it's simply there and it's what we create around it that makes it good or bad in our minds. It's surrounded by standards. Whether you're brought up in a religious, secular or hippie home there are expectations and standards communicated verbally and by example all around. We take on these standards naturally and begin to believe they are right without testing them.

Then, we start to explore our sexuality, we start to get into relationships and discover that not everyone has the same feelings and standards around sex. We may also discover that what we've learned is becoming a little confusing because it doesn't match with reality. And then add some overwhelm and disenchantment with the way our lives are going and it's no wonder that we close down or give little attention to our sexual side.

THE BAD KITTY'S TAIL:

As mentioned before, I grew up in a church going home. I was inundated with messages about no sex before marriage, the dirtiness or sex, the practicality of sex, that sexy clothing was wrong, that being a sexual being – other than for procreation – was wrong. I got other messages from my mom who made no bones about the fact that she loved sex. Every other kid I knew was mortified by the prospect of their parents having sex and was pretty sure they never did it. There was no doubt my mom did. In that sense, I grew up with a healthier attitude than my buds.

I did grow up naive, despite my mom's willingness to talk about sex and her sex life. In grade 12 a friend told a joke about a blow job. I laughed with everyone else but had no idea what it was. I didn't have my first boyfriend – and first kiss – until I was 19.

After a year of fighting the urge with boyfriend number one, I finally had sex and it was like a light went on for me. WOW! In retrospect, it was bad sex, but it was something I wanted to have more. So began the clash of my desire and my need to be a good girl and follow all the rules.

Due to this struggle, I made a lot of bad decisions and spent a lot of time feeling guilty and worried about consequences. I made bad boyfriend choices because whether they were interested in me was the main criteria. I married too young to a man that wasn't a good fit so I could have sex without guilt.

It took a long time for me to really grasp my sexuality, which meant I had to tap into my sensuality first. Now, my sexuality is an integral and integrated part of me. I'm clear on what I need – and what I don't, like marriage. I'm clear on what I like. I'm more willing to try new things. I'm no longer embarrassed by being sexual. I'm comfortable in my body and although it's far from perfect, I love being naked. I've discovered that I'm bi and love women almost as much as men. I like groups, BDSM and anal. All of these things I wouldn't have even considered had I stayed stuck in the standards of others. And oh how much pleasure I would have missed!

Without knowing your full expression through Authentic Sensuality, you may be putting on a false Sexuality. My authentic sexuality is different than yours. Like all other areas of your life, you need to be clear on whom you are, what you want and communicate it effectively in order to live authentically.

When I see people come out to clubs and sit in a corner until they've had a few to become "comfortable" with flirting and dirty dancing I know that that is not their authenticity. It may be part of them, but they have not come to a place that they can express it honestly yet. They still feel they need a little extra courage. Until you can express your desires in all areas of your life, especially sexually, straight and unencumbered by manufactured confidence, you aren't Authentic.

BAD KITTY SCRATCHING POST:

Take a moment with your notebook.

List the standards you grew up with regarding sex. Go through them and cross off ones you have already determined don't work for you. Put a question mark beside the ones you're unsure of. Highlight the ones that you know work in your life.

How many of them are highlighted? Move those onto another page and add to them. What are the things that you have discovered that really work for you around the subject of sex. What do you enjoy? What do you believe? What would you like to explore?

Remember to live only by your standards. Keep your list in mind and when something comes up that doesn't work for you, be honest about it with yourself first and with others if necessary. And, especially start trying those ones that you'd like to explore but haven't yet. Open new doors for yourself.

There are so many aspects to Sexuality. Have

fun with it. Explore, be in the moment. Like every-thing else in your life, it's simply a part of your full expression. Until you allow it to be real for you, you cannot be fully Authentic in your Sensuality.

The way you talk to people, the way you dress, how you flirt, it's all part of it. Do it the way that works for you and enjoy! Live in the moment. Be beautiful in your Sexuality.

Remember, your Authentic Sensuality is how you are in every situation, with every person, in every moment. It may take some time to discover your Authenticity in each moment. The important thing is that you're seeking and looking and doing. Like everything, it's a process. It will come easier to FEEL all aspects of yourself. To SENSE what works and what doesn't; to truly KNOW yourself and live in that place. Go ahead, you gorgeous thing – be you!

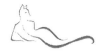

CHAPTER EIGHT:

WHERE DOES THE BAD KITTY GO NOW?

It's been a fun journey – discovering where you've been holding back your Authentic Sensuality, building it back up and expressing it in all areas of your life, including sexually. You may be thinking, but now what?

One of the things that may happen is that not everyone is going to like the "new" but actually old you. The real you that had been buried for so long, it now looks like this new person that those who have known you for years don't recognize. Family can be especially hard in this case.

THE BAD KITTY'S TAIL:

I've talked a lot about how the expectations of what my family thought I was created a lot of tension for me in trying to be what I thought I should be rather than who I am.

For the most part, I've been lucky. My sister, who I'm closest to, has accepted and even encouraged my growth and change. She doesn't always understand some of the courses and things that I'm doing, but she doesn't try to make me go backwards.

My mom is, for the most part, accepting. However, I do get the occasional "What happened to my good little church girl?" comment. My mom probably knows the least about what I have explored, simply because she is the least likely to really get it. She sees the results, but doesn't know that much about how I got there.

I don't have a lot of friends for life. Since we moved a lot, I'm not one of those people that still have the same friends I had in elementary school. Many of the friends I did have when I was a younger adult don't fit in with my growth path. Many of them are negative or stuck. Others are simply not open to new ideas. They have slowly drifted away. I rarely hear from anyone I knew before I started to learn and grow and change back to my true self. Thankfully those few "friends" have been replaced by people who understand the evolving me, are positive, love a challenge and share similar values.

The cool thing is that I now have more, and better, friends than I ever did before.

ANOTHER BAD KITTY'S TAIL:

But what about people that don't have it so easy? What about those whose families reject them, whose spouses leave them, whose kids won't talk to them, who end up friendless?

First of all, let's address that story head on. Realize this – it's a story. It's a fear in your head that is holding you back. No one loses everyone from their lives. I can almost guarantee that some will leave, and I can also guarantee that you probably don't want them around in the long run anyway. Still, I do understand that losing people can be hard.

A woman, *Maggie, was on a growth path. She was tired of feeling lost and directionless. She was sick of feeling alone in a roomful of people. She was finished with being afraid to open her mouth because of fear. She hated being negative about virtually everything. In her late 50's, she was ready for a radical do-over on her life.

One reason she hadn't taken this step sooner was due to her husband. They had been married over 20 years and had three children together. In general he was a good man. He had supported the family well, allowing her to stay home when the children were young. He was never abusive. He did, however, like to keep Maggie where she was. He didn't like change. When she announced she wanted to get a job after all the children were older, he did everything he could to keep her home, from bribery to anger. Eventually, she did get a part time job with a non-profit environmental organization she respected. In essence, it didn't change anything about the running of the household – she was still home to make dinner every day and still did everything she had always done. However, she did feel happier and more fulfilled. Still, it took her husband over a year to accept this change, somewhat begrudgingly.

When Maggie informed him she wanted to start exploring some personal growth courses he strongly objected. He even got the kids on board to make coercive arguments against the entire industry. It got so overwhelming for her that she started taking them on the sly. She would make up stories about having to go take care of a friend or visiting family in order to get away for the occasional evening or weekend.

Soon it became impossible to hide that something was happening. Things began to shift. She rediscovered her passion for the environment – as more than a paper pusher – and wanted to start a recycling program in her small community. Her family was flabbergasted. All of a sudden their quiet, always-at-home wife and mom was out canvassing the neighbourhood and talking to city officials and big business. What was going on?! They didn't like it one bit.

To Maggie's credit, she didn't let the actions of her family stop her. She continued on. Eventually, her husband made the ultimate threat – if you keep doing this, I'm leaving. He simply couldn't handle the changes in her. He wanted his quiet, subservient wife back. This cut her to the core. No matter how much it hurt, she knew if she went backwards she would become bitter and the relationship may end anyway. She explained – once again – why this was important to her and if he couldn't support her, then maybe he should go. He did. One of her children stopped talking to her for several years as well. Of the few friends she had, some were frightened by the changes they saw, others were in awe, many stopped coming by for tea or calling at all. Being in a small community, this was especially hard. When you run into an old friend at the grocery store and they walk by like you're not there, it's hard to take.

Maggie continued on her path of growth. She succeeded in getting the recycling program going and expanded it to include other communities. She made great friends who understood, respected and loved her. Her child eventually started communicating again and is now taking one of the courses that got Maggie motivated. She hasn't remarried. She is dating. She does miss her husband at times. She doesn't miss feeling stuck and lost.

I, and you, have no way of knowing if your experience will be more like mine or Maggie's. You may be telling yourself that it'll be much worse! "I'll lose everything! No one will ever talk to me again. My family will hate me." One thing I can assure you is it won't be as bad as you think. We are so good at making up these crazy stories in our heads about how scary or difficult something is going to be and, in my experience; they never live up to our story.

There will be some challenges along the way, of course. So how do you handle it? The simple answer is, remain true to yourself. You are discovering your Authentic Sensuality as you go. Use the tools you've been using so far in every situation. Take the time to breathe. Use the Axioms. Identify your filters. Use that handy notebook. Be in the moment and observe what's happening.

BAD KITTY SCRATCHING POST:

As you go along, fear will come up. The game we love to play with ourselves – What If – will want your attention repeatedly.
- What if I lose my job?
- What if my husband leaves me?
- What if my parents think I'm crazy?
  What if my friends hate me?

When the What Ifs come up, play a new game with yourself. The "What's the Worst Thing" game.

For each fear, speculate about what's the absolute worst thing that could happen as a result. Take the job loss. Keep asking – What's the worst thing that could happen?

- What's the worst thing that could happen? If I lose my job, I'll feel like a loser.

- What's the worst thing that could happen? If I feel like a loser I'll get depressed.
- What's the worst thing that could happen? If I get depressed I won't be motivated to find a new job.
- What's the worst thing that could happen? If I'm not motivated I won't have any income.
- What's the worst thing that could happen? If I don't have any income, I won't be able to pay my bills.
- What's the worst thing that could happen? If I can't pay my bills I'll be out on the street.
- What's the worst thing that could happen? If I'm out on the street I might start doing drugs or turning tricks.
- What's the worst thing that could happen? If I start doing drugs or turning tricks I might get really sick.
- What's the worst thing that could happen? If I get really sick, I might die.

The purpose of this exercise is to give some perspective. We let our fears get so big in our heads when if we actually looked at them we'd see that they're pretty ridiculous and the worst thing is almost always not going to happen. In fact, over a short span of time, the opposite is likely to happen. So why not play the other side of the coin as well. "What's the Best Thing" game.

If I lose my job:

- What's the best thing that could happen? If I lose my job, I might get over my feelings of malaise and depression.
- What's the best thing that could happen? If I lose my job, I might find an even better one.

- What's the best thing that could happen? If I lose my job, I might have a chance to start that business I've always wanted.
- What's the best thing that could happen? If I lose my job, I might have a great extended vacation.
- What's the best thing that could happen? If I lose my job, I might discover my true passion.
- What's the best thing that could happen? If I lose my job, I might be a lot happier.
- What's the best thing that could happen? If I lose my job, I might find another way to make even better money.
- What's the best thing that could happen? If I lose my job, I might be able to spend more time with my family.
- What's the best thing that could happen? If I lose my job, I might have time to do the (fill in the blank) that I've always wanted.

Chances are very good, now that you're living a more aware and authentic life, that the best things will happen rather than the worst. Isn't it worth going through the fear to find that "best things" place?

THE UNKNOWN:

Ok, sure, but losing a job is one thing. Having people in your family never talk to you again or your husband leave you is another. Really, it only feels different. In the end it's all the same. Change is hard and very few of us like it. Patterns and familiarity are good to have. They make us feel safe, even if they're not healthy.

Ask any woman who's ever left an abusive relationship. For those of us on the outside it looks like a no-brainer. He's hitting you – get out! On the inside it's much harder. Even in the pain there's a sense of safety because it's familiar. What's out there is the scary part. It's the "What next?" the unknown, that strikes fear in our hearts. No matter what our situation is, it's the fear of the unknown that keeps us where we are.

That's why the above exercise is so helpful. It puts some clarity on the best and worst scenarios. No matter what the situation is, chances are, if you feel the push for a change, there's a reason. Yes, you may feel very comfortable with your husband. You may have built a life together. And now that you've made some changes in your life, you're feeling held back. He's not supporting you emotionally anymore. There's a sense of resentment building on both sides. You have a decision to make – can you remain Authentically Sensual in this situation or do you need to move away to keep yourself?

Your mom loves you. But she really loved the "old" you. Every time you talk to her she brings up how she doesn't like the way you've changed. She doesn't like that you left your job. She thinks your new business idea is crazy. Every time you leave her you feel small, beaten down and it takes you several days to rebound. You can't disown your mom – or whatever family member it may be. Well, I suppose you can, but most of us would rather not. You have a decision to make. How much time do you spend with her? How do you steer the conversation? What do you do to prepare and buffer yourself so you feel stronger rather than weaker when you leave?

Remember, you always have a choice, in every situation. I can't – and won't from these pages – tell you what's the best thing to do. It's all individual. There are no hard and fast rules. You are living Authentically now, only you know the right answer. I – or someone else – can certainly guide you to those answers through coaching. In the end, you know the right answer. Trust yourself. Use the tools you've been developing and figure it out!

THE BAD KITTY'S TAIL:

Before I started The Bad Kitty, I was working with a party plan company. It was through this company that I started instructing pole dancing. The company went through several transitions over the four years I was with them. Each change was designed to make the company more viable over the long term and to make more money for the women involved.

I experienced the opposite. My income went down and I felt less and less congruence between my goals and those of the company. I understood intellectually why they were making the changes. My gut said they didn't work. For me. One thing that wasn't working was that they were putting less and less emphasis on the pole dancing part of the business. So much so that by the last year there was no mention of it on the website.

After about 6 months of hemming and hawing, being unhappy and thinking that I could make it work no matter what because I loved the people who started the company, I started to create The Bad Kitty. As the ball started to gently roll, things started to come into place. My vision got clearer all the time. The website came together like a dream. I was given the name. I found someone who created the perfect logo. Everyone who has seen me struggle over the years to figure out my passion and direction saw something new and solid in me. This was the project that was my Authentic Self.

After building The Bad Kitty for 8 months, things were starting the come together. I was nearly done the first draft of this book. I had done some of my new programs. I had gotten my first big speaking engagement. Then the news came via email.

The company I had been working with was going out of business. I guess I wasn't the only one the changes didn't fit with! It wasn't a big surprise, but it was sad. I respect the people who started the business and they had a great passion for it. Unfortunately all the changes turned people off; they slowly drifted away and the owners never did manage to rebuild the momentum.

I did what was right for me. I felt bad because I wanted to be loyal to these people that I had come to care about and who had done so much for me. In the end, I had to do what was right for me and it turned out to be a really good idea! If I had waited until the business folded, I may not have had the energy or desire to create what I had created.

Everything happened in the timing it was supposed to. I learned a lot from being involved in that company. It was all perfect – ups and downs and all.

Every situation that comes your way has a positive side. All we have to do is look for it. It isn't always immediately apparent, but it will come to be.

THE BAD KITTY'S TAIL:

After my marriage, my next big relationship turned into a live in situation. We were together for 5 years. It's a funny thing about relationships; each time you up the level of commitment, a small piece of your armour comes off and you become more Authentic. It isn't intentional, it's just human nature. Think back to how you are on a first date versus after you've been with someone for some time. It's very different. It's not that we necessarily hide anything on purpose; it's simply how we're built.

For me, the higher the level of commitment, the more I get comfortable. I stop making as much of an effort. I think that's the same for many of us. *Ron and I are well matched and we're still good friends. Unfortunately, what we need in a relationship is different. I wasn't providing what he needed in a way that worked for him so he sought it elsewhere and had an affair.

When I discovered he had been cheating for nearly a year with a much younger woman – how cliché – I was, of course, devastated. How could anyone cheat on me? I love sex. I'm willing to try new things. I'm hot! But that wasn't enough. He needed something I wasn't providing and possibly would never be able to do because of who I am, no matter how much I may have tried.

The relationship ended. There was plenty of animosity, especially from me, for some time. Eventually we became friends again. That is a positive on its own. In addition, it was after this break up that I really started to explore possibilities for myself and my future. I discovered the pole dancing company. I managed an apartment building that went condo, bought a suite, renovated and flipped it with the help of incredible friends and family and bought my house. I started The Bad Kitty. I discovered that I love being on my own.

If we were still together, it's unlikely that many of these results would have occurred. A time of intense pain and recrimination turned out to be one of the best events of my life!

ANOTHER BAD KITTY'S TAIL:

A man had a passion. It was an unusual passion that wouldn't make him any money, but he pursued it anyway. His passion was self help books. He quit his job and started to read. It's all he did. He felt that if he pursued his passion, everything else in life would simply take care of itself.

After some time his savings started to run out and he found it hard to buy groceries. Around that time he started to get many invitations for meals with friends and others. People found him fascinating to talk to because of all the knowledge he was amassing and liked to have him around.

Not long after this, his accounts got really low and he was about to lose his home. He was prepared to be homeless if he could still pursue his passion. Instead people started asking him to housesit. He sold his possessions and became a nomad, living in house after house for weeks or months at a time. The whole time he continued to read, absorb and integrate.

Eventually the news of his diverse knowledge and interest spread and he began to get requests to speak. He is now an international speaker who doesn't have to rely on dinners out or house sitting to get by. His passion turned into a lucrative and fulfilling business.

Yes, this is an extreme story. The point is, it may take some time, but there is always something positive. Follow your dreams, know yourself, live your passion and you will see results! Always look for the good in yourself, in others, in your situation. It's always there, somewhere.

BAD KITTY SCRATCHING POST:

One more time with your notebook:

Think of a time that was hard in your life. Write it down in detail. What has happened since? What positive things have happened as a result? Write it down in detail.

Read it aloud. Feel the difficult emotions that may re-emerge. Feel the sense of gratitude and excitement at what has come as a result. Celebrate the latter. Do a happy dance. Push an Easy Button. Hoot and holler. Recognize how far you've come!

Living your Authentic Sensuality is easy – and not so easy:
- Be gentle with yourself; life can get hard. You will experience setbacks. Know that it's all part of the process.
- Celebrate your success.
- Be easy on yourself in your struggles.
- Recognize the stories that you tell yourself. Are they serving you or destroying you?
- Speak up for yourself.
- Be present at all times.
- Act in spite of fear.
- Look to your Sensual heroes. Use chapter 3 for examples.
- Remember what makes you happy, what

drives you and live by it.

- Share your passion with the world.
- Do what satisfies you first.
- Keep your tank full!
- Take plenty of me time.
- Be aware of your patterns and filters. Use the ones that serve you, discard the ones that don't.
- Above all, love yourself.

You are so amazing. As you discover more and more about yourself as you go along your journey, you will realize just how amazing you are.

You are lovable.

You are worthy.

You are YOU!

Thank you for being you. Your light shines brightly in the world. Keep it out there for all to see. BE BEAUTIFUL, my dear, BE YOU.

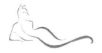

THE FINAL BAD KITTY BIG MEOW

You've come a long way, baby! I hope that you've been celebrating along the way. It's so easy to forget where we've come from and only see how far we still think we need to go.

Celebrate every step. Look back and see how far you've come down the road before looking to the next step.

Set your sights on where you want to go and remember you're already on the way. Every step, no matter how small it may seem is a victory.

BAD KITTY SCRATCHING POST:

You deserve this.

Go to the mirror. Full length preferred. Naked is best. Set a timer for 5 minutes. Spend the 5 minutes alone with yourself in the mirror. Do nothing else. No make up application. No brushing your teeth. If the phone rings and you answer it, start over. Do 5 UNINTERRUPTED minutes.

Look at yourself. Go back over what you've learned in your journey with THE BAD KITTY HANDBOOK. Think about the activities you've done. Think about the successes you've had. Look at yourself as you do this. Celebrate the beauty you see in the mirror. Recognize how undeniably gorgeous you are, just as you are.

At the end of the 5 minutes, look yourself in the

eye and say, "You are incredible. You deserve every-thing you want. You deserve to be cared for. You deserve the very best. You are beautiful. I love you!"

Go into the world, my kitties. Go and spread the word about how wonderful every woman you meet is. Tell others about their beauty because chances are, they don't see it. Share your joy, your passion, yourself with everyone. Be brave.

I simply can't say it enough – BE BEAUTIFUL, BE YOU! You are all my heroes.

Love you all,

Christie Mawer

The Bad Kitty
www.thebadkitty.com
Christie@thebadkitty.com
Edmonton, Alberta Canada

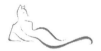

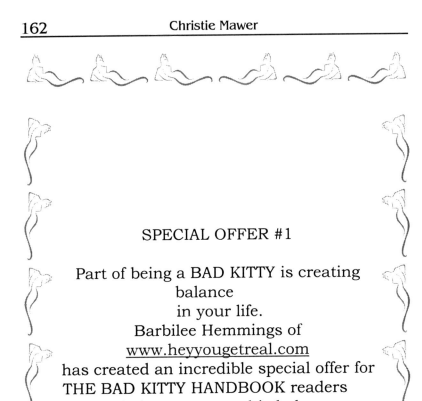

SPECIAL OFFER #1

Part of being a BAD KITTY is creating
balance
in your life.
Barbilee Hemmings of
www.heyyougetreal.com
has created an incredible special offer for
THE BAD KITTY HANDBOOK readers
to help you create this balance
in your finances and health.

Go to
www.heyyougetreal.com/thebadkitty
and you will receive
BOTH of Barbilee's ebooks for FREE!!!

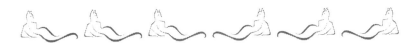

SPECIAL OFFER #2

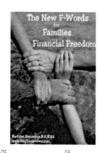
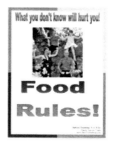

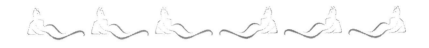

SPECIAL OFFER #3

Continue your BAD KITTY journey
with 2 ebooks
full of tips for staying in touch with
your Authentic Sensuality.

Go to http://beingsensual.com/prod-
ucts.html
Enter coupon code HANDBOOK and
receive
both ebooks for FREE!

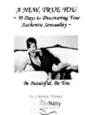

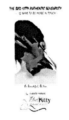

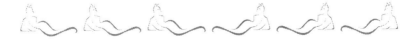

SPECIAL OFFER #4

Contact Christie, THE BAD KITTY for your personal and private SENSUALITY COACHING.

<u>PACKAGE ONE - THE HOUSECAT:</u>

6 Sessions, one half hour every other week. One on one, over the phone. Designed to give you the tools to understand who you are, what you want and how to express it Authentically in every situation. YOUR SENSUALITY COACH will keep you accountable, offer suggestions and reveal patterns that may be holding you back. This is a start and will bring out much of your inner BAD KITTY.

<u>PACKAGE TWO – THE BOBCAT:</u>

9 Sessions, one half hour every other week. One on one session over the phone and webcam or Skype. Designed to give you the tools of package one in addition to evaluating your body language, facial expressions and dress. This package will take you deeper, get you in your body and bring your dreams more into focus. It will give you tools to move forward toward your ideal life.

<u>PACKAGE THREE - THE BIG CAT:</u>

12 Sessions, one half hour every week. One on one session over the phone and by webcam or Skype. This more concentrated package will move you along faster, challenge you more deeply and push your buttons. It will give you the will, tools and desire to really make things happen that you've been wanting in your life. Dance will be incorporated in these sessions.

Email <u>Christie@thebadkitty.com</u> and use the subject line HANDBOOK COACHING to receive $100 off the package of your choice.

SPECIAL OFFER #5

Contact Christie, THE BAD KITTY,
for a
FREE CHAIR DANCING LESSON.

In the privacy of your own home
over Skype or
Webcam, receive a half hour
instruction that will
result in a full routine on the chair
that you can
do anytime, anywhere just for you
or
for someone special.

Sensual dance of all kinds, including chair dancing,
is a great way to stay in touch with
your amazing
Authentic Sensuality and to remind
you

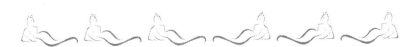

LaVergne, TN USA
07 December 2010
207638LV00006B/2/P

9 780982 575574